REIKI

REIKI

A Comprehensive Guide

PAMELA
MILES

JEREMY P. TARCHER/PENGUIN

a member of Penguin Group (USA) Inc.

New York

JEREMY P. TARCHER/PENGUIN
Published by the Penguin Group
Penguin Group (USA) Inc., 375 Hudson Street, New York, New York 10014, USA • Penguin Group (Canada),
90 Eglinton Avenue East, Suite 700, Toronto, Ontario M4P 2Y3, Canada (a division of Pearson Canada Inc.) •
Penguin Books Ltd, 80 Strand, London WC2R 0RL, England • Penguin Ireland, 25 St Stephen's Green, Dublin 2,
Ireland (a division of Penguin Books Ltd) • Penguin Group (Australia), 250 Camberwell Road, Camberwell, Victoria 3124,
Australia (a division of Pearson Australia Group Pty Ltd) • Penguin Books India Pvt Ltd, 11 Community Centre,
Panchsheel Park, New Delhi–110 017, India • Penguin Group (NZ), 67 Apollo Drive, Rosedale, North Shore 0632,
New Zealand (a division of Pearson New Zealand Ltd) • Penguin Books (South Africa) (Pty) Ltd,
24 Sturdee Avenue, Rosebank, Johannesburg 2196, South Africa

Penguin Books Ltd, Registered Offices: 80 Strand, London WC2R 0RL, England

First trade paperback edition 2008
Copyright © 2006 by Pamela Miles
Published simultaneously in Canada

Most Tarcher/Penguin books are available at special quantity discounts for bulk purchase for sales promotions, premiums, fund-raising, and educational needs. Special books or book excerpts also can be created to fit specific needs. For details, write Penguin Group (USA) Inc. Special Markets, 375 Hudson Street, New York, NY 10014.

The Library of Congress catalogued the hardcover as follows:

Miles, Pamela, date.
Reiki : a comprehensive guide / Pamela Miles.
p.   cm.
Includes index.
ISBN 1-58542-474-9
ISBN 978-1-58542-649-2 (paperback edition)
1. Reiki (Healing system).   2. Alternative medicine.   3. Integrative medicine.   I. Title.
RZ403.R45   2006   2005054881
615.8'51—dc22

Printed in the United States of America
1   3   5   7   9   10   8   6   4   2

Book design by Meighan Cavanaugh

Illustrations by Retsu Takahashi

To my mother,

and to all who seek to

nourish and to serve

CONTENTS

ACKNOWLEDGMENTS

Writing a book is a study in contrasts, a process both solitary and collaborative, and, in this case, one with a long story of its own. I have more people to thank than pages on which to do it. To each of you who have supported Reiki and this project by sharing your Reiki stories, explaining your work, making introductions, and generally giving encouragement: We both know who you are. I remember you often, with warm gratitude. Thank you to my clients and students for sharing yourselves, your insights, and your experiences. And a special thank-you to the many scientists who generously and patiently explained your work to me, even though many of you had never heard of Reiki. Your contribution has been invaluable to the development of this book and to my continuing education.

Speaking with friends and colleagues in both conventional health care and traditional healing arts and spirituality is not only a delightful way to spend time, but a treasured source of stimulation and education. Heartfelt thanks to Robert Abramson, M.D., M.Ac.; Kausthub Desikachar; Sally (Durgananda) Kempton; Robert Schmehr, CSW; Albert Kuperman, Ph.D.; Larry Dossey, M.D.; Lewis Mehl-Madrona, M.D., Ph.D.; Master Yu Wen Ru; Do-Hyun Choe, OMD; Injae Choe, LMT; Carol Davis, Ph.D.; Danna Doyle Park, M.D.; Donna Eden; David Feinstein, Ph.D.; David Riley, M.D.; Bert Petersen, M.D.; John Friend; Vasant Lad; Lokendra Singh; Kenneth Cohen; Kumiko Kanayama; David Crow, L.Ac.; Pankaj Naram; Simon Taffler; Rubin Naiman, Ph.D.; Melinda Mingus, M.D.; Leslie Kaminoff; Michael Cohen, Esq.; Joel Friedman, M.D., Ph.D.; and Lawrence Palevsky, M.D. Special thanks to Andrew Weil, M.D., for your support of subtle healing therapies and your leadership in both medical and consumer education.

The ongoing conversation with my Reiki colleagues continually inspires me and moves my understanding to greater clarity and refinement. Huge thanks to Barbara McDaniel; Robert Fueston, L.Ac.; Paul Prakash Dennis; Linda Keiser Mardis; Wendy Miner, LMT.; Elaine Abrams; and Nancy Eos, M.D.

Thank you to my colleagues who learned Reiki from Hawayo Takata and carry her work forth with such commitment, devotion, and humility: Wanja Twan, Paul Mitchell, Susan Mitchell, Rick Bockner, Anneli Twan, and Chelsea Van Koughnett.

I extend deep gratitude to my esteemed Japanese colleagues, Reiki masters Hyakuten Inamoto and Hiroshi Doi, for your availability and patience as I tested the accuracy of my information and the subtlety of my understanding, and to Toshihiko Murata for your gracious translation and perceptive dialogue. Thank you, Phyllis Lei Furumoto, for your kind permission to include the photos of Mikao Usui, Chujiro Hayashi, and your grandmother, Hawayo Takata.

The vision of two key people moved this book from dream to reality: my agent, Stephanie Kip Rostan, and the publisher of Tarcher, Joel Fotinos. My editor, Ashley Shelby, extended herself far beyond the call of duty to craft the manuscript, and deftly coordinated Tarcher's stellar Team Reiki: managing editor Amy Brosey, designer Meighan Cavanaugh, jacket designer Lee Fukui, and copy editors Barbara Grenquist and Anna Jardine. And thank you, Retsu Takahashi, for your commitment and care in illustrating the hand placements.

As the manuscript developed, I pressed colleagues and friends for edit after edit after edit. For your dialogue, your indulgence, your thoughtful perspective that shaped this manuscript, and your love of the practice, I thank Sheldon Lewis; Susie Kessler; Michael Gnatt, M.D.; Sezelle Haddon, M.D.; Ben Kligler, M.D.; Indrani Weber; Judith Jacobson, Ph.D.; Tess Nakamura; Sheila Lewis; and MaryAnn Zitka. And thank you to Rosemarie Turk, Philip Baloun, Nurit Spector, Dafna Schmerin, and the remaining members of the board of the Institute for the Advancement of Complementary Therapies (I*ACT), Norman Solovay, Mackie Davis, and Alma Montclair, for your friendship and support.

Throughout my life, I have been tremendously fortunate to be mentored by accomplished teachers of many wisdom traditions: you have all left your vibration in my heart. Many years ago, Lama Thubten Yeshe and Lama Zopa Rinpoche provided my first glimpse of living compassion. More recently, His Holiness Orygen Kusum Lingpa has immeasurably deepened my understanding of healing and spirituality. The teachings and Healing Chod offered by Dungse Rigdzin Dorje Rinpoche and the lamas and nuns of Zangdokpalri Monastery have been a source of profound support and a reminder of the connection between healing and self-determination.

This book could never have happened without the blessings, teachings, and unfailing example of the Siddha Yoga lineage of meditation masters, Gurumayi Chidvilasanda, Swami Muktananda, and Bhagawan Nityananda, who continually reveal to me the sweet transformation that comes with practice and grace.

To my children, Eric and Hannah Grace: You are, alas, children no longer. Thank you for the inspiration and sheer delight of being your mother.

FOREWORD

Reiki is a system of healing and spiritual development that has enjoyed substantial popularity and success worldwide. With that popularity have come some challenges that this book ably addresses through an informed historical, clinical, and scientific perspective and a mature vision for Reiki's continuing evolution. Originating in Japan nearly a century ago, the practice has been taught to millions of people. But, like many Western transplants from Eastern traditions, it has become seriously diluted at its most popularized fringes, with large numbers of individuals, for instance, becoming "Reiki masters" after three weekends of training or less.

Miles makes a vivid case that Reiki is well worth liberating from these devolving standards, not through increased regulation, but through deepened understanding. At the most basic level, she recounts how physicians she has trained report that hands-on Reiki "bridges the gap that can exist between touch that is investigative and touch that is therapeutic." The approach reacquaints us, in our high-tech/low-touch society, with the healing power of loving, supportive, nonsexual physical contact and offers a graceful context for offering it. At the most profound level, as conventional medicine wrestles with the implications of the convergences among quantum physics, superstring theory ("vibration is everything"), and frontier topics in biomedical research such as cell regeneration and the human biofield, Reiki may be way ahead of the curve in showing how the emerging paradigm can be applied in health-care settings and for self-healing.

The fundamentals of Reiki can indeed be transmitted in as little as eight to ten hours. That is among Reiki's greatest strengths. People can be practicing it on themselves and their friends after a weekend class or short series of evening sessions. And they can do this responsibly. A Reiki session is at least as safe as a gentle massage. If people can practice Reiki responsibly and safely after just a brief course, the next question is, "Does it work?" What can actually be delivered after only a day's training in a practice whose advocates claim has such breadth and depth?

My background is in energy medicine. I teach my students to assess energy imbalances systematically and to intervene actively. The path taken in Reiki is more receptive than active, more like meditation than medicine. Reiki is generally associated with "nonspecific" benefits—such as deep relaxation, stress reduction, more restful sleep, enhanced immune functioning, greater peace, and increased self-awareness—rather than with the treatment of specific illnesses (though these nonspecific benefits can have a strong impact on an illness). While these benefits can be attributed to features common to any healing modality, such as the practitioner's caring or the recipient's hunger for touch or belief that something positive is about to happen, Miles makes the case that something more profound is occurring.

Reiki is the name of the practice, but it is also the name of the pervasive spirit or "sacred pulsation" that is purportedly the basis of the practice. In Japanese, *Rei* means universal, often with the connotation of a "Universal Intelligence." *Ki* means a "nonphysical energy" that also entails a sacred connotation, perhaps closer to the holy atmosphere one might experience at a regal mountaintop, a shrine, or other sacred site than an energy that can be measured by gross physical instruments. And it is here that Reiki further breaks away from conventional scientific frameworks, for this universal pulsation is accessed through initiations, sacred symbols, and distant treatment.

But before we discount too rapidly these ideas and practices that are so foreign to our culture (though consistent with the worldview and traditions of the country where the practice originated), we need to recognize the growing support for such ideas even within conventional scientific frameworks. For instance, one of the published peer-reviewed studies that support the efficacy of Reiki which Miles cites investigated its effects on depression. Participants who scored high on standard depression scales received hands-on Reiki treatments for six weeks and improved significantly more than participants who received a placebo treatment (and tests a year later showed that the benefits held, even though no additional treatment was offered). But a third group within this study received "distant Reiki," a form of the approach that can be administered from another location. While conventional science has no explanation yet for such practices, just as we lack coherent scientific explanations for the documented healing effects of prayer in behalf of individuals who are ill, the group that received "distant Reiki" showed improvements that were equivalent to those receiving hands-on Reiki. Clearly, since studies of this nature have been rapidly accumulating in recent years, concepts that transcend our Newtonian time-space models are needed, and Reiki is one that has both history and practical results behind it.

I agree with the author that Reiki is worthy of serious attention as a viable health-care practice and as a way of probing the larger dimensions of the story we are all living. And I admire the clear, straightforward, yet penetrating way this superb book addresses the issues that those interested in exploring Reiki, as well as those already well versed in the approach, would want to understand. *Reiki: A Comprehensive Guide* will prove to be a great contribution to the practice, dissemination, and creative evolution of this easily accessed yet ultimately profound technique.

Donna Eden
November 2005
Ashland, Oregon

INTRODUCTION

I came upon Reiki in the throes of first-trimester pregnancy blahs. A friend offered me some relief. I jumped at the chance, and landed on a springboard that catapulted me into the rest of my life. Until I learned Reiki, I was able to trigger healing in my clients, but in spite of (and sometimes it felt like in mockery of) my skill and knowledge, I myself was frequently sick. Nothing serious, but it happened often enough to get in the way and seemed so unnecessary. The irony of my plight did not escape me.

All that frustration changed with a single Reiki treatment. As my friend's hands rested lightly on my head, I was irresistibly drawn to a quiet place deep within while I experienced cascades of pulsations throughout my being. And I mean my being—it wasn't just a physical sensation, although there was a definite physical response. But also, a joyful, refreshing sensation scampered everywhere. By the end of the session I felt profoundly realigned. And wanting to learn more. But I didn't want to learn how Reiki worked—my years of meditation and spiritual practices gave me an awareness of what Reiki was doing and comfort in my direct perception. I wanted to learn to practice Reiki.

And so I did. My friend's Reiki master didn't have a class scheduled soon enough for my enthusiasm, so she offered me private instruction. I was happy not to wait, but found the class itself a bit boring. The Reiki master was lovely, but the explanations she offered seemed neither necessary nor satisfying. I wondered if I had made a mistake.

Then came the first of four initiations, subtle transmissions that empower the student to practice Reiki. Once again I felt the pulsations. Later that day, I began practicing Reiki on myself. I have never stopped.

Since learning to practice Reiki in 1986, I have brought Reiki training and treatment into major New York City hospitals and have taught Reiki to patients and their families; to doctors, nurses, medical students, and other health professionals; and to many people who are healthy and happy and want to stay that way—or be even healthier and happier. I've taught Reiki to people of all ages, from toddlers to a ninety-three-year-old Holocaust survivor. Each one has found his or her unique relationship with Reiki, using it at times and in ways that are individually meaningful. Kids use Reiki to calm themselves before a test and sharpen their focus during it. Parents use Reiki at bedtime—theirs and their kids'. Both competitive athletes and weekend warriors use Reiki to boost stamina and speed recovery from inevitable sports-related injuries. Once you have been trained in Reiki, you can lightly lay your hand on your head, chest, abdomen, or any place that hurts, anytime you need to regain your center, restore your well-being, or relieve pain—even while you're in a cab, or watching TV, or on the phone with your mother-in-law.

Reiki has helped people with chronic pain, heart disease, cancer, HIV, diabetes, depression, trauma, neurodegenerative disorders, fatigue syndromes, infertility, cerebral palsy, recovery from stroke—the list goes on and on. It is used to support conventional medical care, hastening surgical recovery and reducing side effects of radiation and chemotherapy. Reiki can smooth the rough edges of necessary but invasive medical treatments and enable patients to tolerate needed pharmaceuticals, or even to need less medication.

People in good health use Reiki to manage stress and strengthen well-being, finding new levels of confidence and self-acceptance, more harmony in family relationships, and a deeper sense of peace and spiritual connectedness. Whether we are sick or well, seeking or satisfied, receiving conventional medical treatment or relying solely on alternative modalities, Reiki can move us gently and powerfully into a deeper state of balance, and connect us to untapped inner resources.

Reiki is an invitation to wellness. Although Reiki is easily practiced, learning it involves a subtle vibrational transmission (which will be discussed in chapter 4). Even more than being *taught* to practice Reiki, you are *empowered* to practice. Thus you can learn Reiki only from a qualified Reiki master, someone who has undergone training and been empowered to empower others.

What this book can do is help you understand this simple, effective healing practice so you can decide for yourself if you want Reiki treatment or training. You'll get strategies to connect with Reiki resources near you, and guidance in choosing the Reiki practitioner who is most qualified and best suited to work with you. And once you have trained with a Reiki master, this book will help guide you on your Reiki journey.

Perhaps you are already a Reiki master, maybe even one who is collaborating in conventional medical environments.* I honor your work and wish to support it. You may find that some of the language in this book is different from yours, but if you have practiced Reiki regularly over a period of years, you will recognize our common experience.

This is not *The Reiki Gospel According to Pamela,* nor is it *The Reiki Rule Book,* but simply a Reiki companion.

There is not one way. In these pages, I share the path I am traveling in the hope that it will enrich your journey.

---

*In this book, the terms "conventional medicine" and "biomedicine" refer to scientific medicine, whereas the terms "traditional medicine," "indigenous medicine," "holistic medicine," and "natural medicine" refer to medical approaches that have come out of healing traditions.

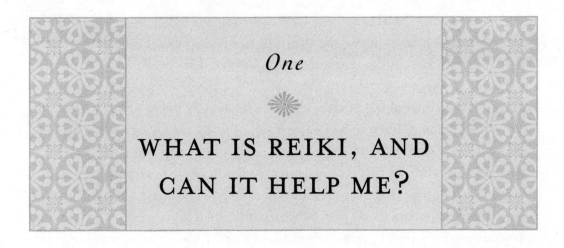

One

WHAT IS REIKI, AND CAN IT HELP ME?

Better than medicine is care of the health.

JAPANESE PROVERB

You are lying fully clothed on a treatment table. As the Reiki practitioner places her hands lightly on your head, you feel yourself drawn into a sweet repose. Her hands eventually move from your head to the front of your torso. You notice that sometimes her hands feel warm, even hot, and deeply soothing. Each hand placement brings a sense of ease into another part of your body, and the busyness of your mind gracefully opens to an inner quiet. She asks you to turn over, and her hands on your back bring yet another sensation of comfort. *You feel you could lie here contentedly for a very long time. . . .*

Just a year ago, Jerry* had been through two grueling heart surgeries within eighteen hours. Now he was returning to the same OR to receive a new heart. But this time, I would be with him in the operating room, offering him hands-on Reiki healing throughout his surgery.

In spite of what lay ahead of him, Jerry was amazingly upbeat. He attributed his steadiness to the confidence he had in his medical team, the loving care of his wife, and to our Reiki sessions. Jerry had not been so upbeat when I was initially called to offer him Reiki after his first two surgeries. At that time, he was quite agitated and struggling in the cardiac intensive-care unit after being in a coma for a week. My hands filled with warm pulsations as I placed them lightly on his head to offer Reiki healing. A few minutes later, Jerry opened his eyes and grinned at me just as he was doing now.

Jerry's improvement was rapid after that treatment, and he was moved out of the intensive-care unit two days later. He continued receiving Reiki in the hospital once or twice a week until his discharge two months later. Jerry felt Reiki strengthened him. His wife found that the mini-treatments I offered her made her less anxious and helped her sleep more soundly.

Although this was the first time I'd attended Jerry during surgery, it was one of many medical procedures I'd taken part in over the years, working with the growing number of physicians and surgeons who have come to recognize the healing potential of Reiki.

As Jerry slowly regained consciousness after transplant surgery, his first thought was "Oh, I guess I didn't get the heart after all." He knew well enough the pain of awakening after heart surgery, but this time was different—so different, in fact, that Jerry didn't need to take any pain medication after this surgery. I continued to offer him Reiki as he recovered from the operation with surprising speed, and before they left the hospital, I trained Jerry and his wife to give themselves (and each other) Reiki at home. Although there is always the risk that the body will reject the new heart, Jerry's two post-op biopsies showed no signs of rejection. The heart surgery saved his life and Reiki helped him heal.

---

*Names and identifying details have been changed to protect the privacy of clients.

"Did I really make my headache go away?" Miguel asked, as my class for HIV out-patients at Beth Israel Medical Center in New York City finished giving themselves their first Reiki treatment. This decorated Vietnam vet had a painful past—a traumatic time in the military, a long term in prison, heroin addiction, and AIDS. Now out of prison and trying to stay clean, he had come to the class to learn Reiki self-treatment. Many of his complaints—fatigue, diarrhea, pain, agitation, insomnia, and migraines—resisted treatment by conventional medications, and he came to class hoping Reiki could help.

Miguel attended the four sessions of Reiki training with great interest, expanding his understanding of well-being and how to care for himself with Reiki's light, heal-ing touch. Giving himself Reiki, he felt, was not just helping his migraines—he sensed something deeper was happening. "I feel hopeful," he said simply. I encouraged him to give himself Reiki consistently, every day.

Several months later, I ran into Miguel in front of Beth Israel. He was still giving himself Reiki daily—sometimes several times a day—and he was no longer getting migraines. Although his roommate had died that very morning, Miguel was remark-ably composed as he expressed gratitude for Reiki's healing presence in his life.

Carolyn was a hard worker who loved her job as a high-level TV producer. One of those people who seems to thrive on stress, this high-spirited blonde worked out reg-ularly, ate well, and enjoyed overall good health—until in her early thirties she lost not one but three pregnancies. With the attention of a skilled and caring high-risk ob-stetrician, Carolyn eventually gave birth to a healthy baby girl. Several years later, during her second anxiety-filled high-risk pregnancy, she came for Reiki treatment and experienced a sense of serenity and well-being she didn't know was possible. After our first session, Carolyn was typically decisive: "I want another appointment next week," she announced, "and I want to learn to practice Reiki on myself and my family." She signed up for my next class.

Once back at work after giving birth to her second child with relative ease, Carolyn stopped coming for sessions, relying on her own hands for her Reiki. Years later, when she unexpectedly became pregnant again at age forty-one, Carolyn returned for treatment. Although her physician expected another high-risk pregnancy, he soon determined the pregnancy was normal. Carolyn went on to have (mostly) natural childbirth in the hospital birthing room, with her husband—and her Reiki master (me)—by her side.

The anecdotal reports of response to Reiki treatment around the world are remarkably similar. These reports come from students who are self-treating, from clients who are receiving treatment from professional Reiki practitioners, and from other people, often health-care providers, who observe the changes that coincide with their patients receiving Reiki treatment. By this time, you are likely wondering what kind of treatment could deliver such wonderful results as those illustrated in the stories above. And, you may be asking, what exactly *is* Reiki?

WHAT IS REIKI?

The simple answer is that Reiki is a spiritual healing practice that can help return us to balanced functioning on every level—physical, mental, emotional, spiritual, even social—regardless of our age or state of health. Although balance can mean different things in different circumstances, Reiki treatment, which is usually facilitated by light touch, typically brings rapid stress reduction and relief from pain and anxiety. Recipients commonly report improved sleep and digestion, and a greater sense of well-being. Other benefits, such as feeling more motivated, less depressed, or experiencing relief from side effects of medications, radiation, or chemotherapy, vary from person to person. Unlike conventional medicine, Reiki does not attack disease. Rather, Reiki supports our well-being and strengthens our natural ability to heal by encouraging balance.

While Reiki treatment can be received from another, Reiki practice is easily learned at the First Degree level and is as effective when offered to oneself as when received from another. Reiki requires no belief, simply the willingness to experience. Noninvasive and holistic, Reiki can be safely practiced in any situation, even emergencies. There are no known medical contraindications.

The National Center for Complementary and Alternative Medicine (NCCAM) of the National Institutes of Health (NIH) classifies Reiki as a form of energy medicine, and specifically a biofield therapy. Biofields are also referred to as putative energy fields because, at this time, there is no technology subtle enough to reproducibly measure biofields in the way scientists can measure magnetic or electrical fields.[1] Biofields are extremely subtle fields that are said to surround and permeate the human body.

Although it makes sense to classify Reiki as energy medicine for research purposes, Reiki really is not energy medicine. That term more accurately refers to such interventions as qigong, shiatsu, or Therapeutic Touch, which deliberately reorganize the biofield, and which require concentration on the part of the practitioner to make a diagnosis, create a treatment plan, and then implement treatment. Reiki is not deliberate in that way. There is no diagnosis. The Reiki practitioner need not concentrate. The practitioner does not direct Reiki. Both the practice and the experience of Reiki are closer to meditation than to any techniques of energy medicine.

In fact, the word *energy,* as vague as it is, does not really apply to Reiki, which is better expressed by more specific and descriptive words such as *pulsation, vibration,* or *oscillation.* Although NCCAM gathers all subtle therapies under one umbrella, putative or biofield therapies, the biofield is actually multileveled, and different therapies address different and distinct levels of subtle reality.

Reiki affects the subtlest level of the biofield, the subtle vibrational body that holds the blueprint for outer, measurable reality. Unlike energy therapies, Reiki is accessed through, but not directed by, the practitioner. Once accessed, Reiki gently encourages the biofield toward balance.

The term *Reiki* is often mistakenly used interchangeably with terms referring to various bioenergies, such *chi* and *prana* (including by NCCAM), but these terms are no more interchangeable than are Chinese medicine and Ayurveda, the systems in which they are described. (Also, there are many types of both chi and prana.) Reiki is much subtler than these bioenergies. It is primordial consciousness,* which is identical to the respective source states of chi and prana, called *yuan chi* (this term can vary among Chinese lineages) and *mahaprana*. The chi manipulated in acupuncture and the prana moved by yogic practices are grosser bioenergies. Chi is just subphysical, but still beyond the reach of technological measurement. Or at least directly. There are measurable changes in electrical conductivity at the site of acupuncture points on the Chinese meridians, the subtle pathways through which chi is said to travel.[2] The presence of such footprints is significant, strengthening the case for the existence of subtle energies while underlining technology's current limitations.

THE LOOK AND FEEL OF REIKI

The hands of a trained Reiki practitioner are placed lightly on a fully clothed recipient who reclines or sits comfortably. When Reiki is offered to someone who is conscious, both practitioner and recipient quickly notice a gentle shift toward relaxation. Breathing becomes slower and more comfortable, and the person may sigh or even snore as the state of relaxation deepens. The experience of Reiki treatment is very subjective and varies from person to person and treatment to treatment. Some recipients feel a warm tingling where Reiki hands are placed, others feel soft waves of subtle pulsations flowing throughout their bodies, and others feel nothing in particular—nothing, except they are very relaxed afterward, with an enhanced sense of well-being. If the person came for treatment with pain, it usually disappears or diminishes during the session. After treatment, the recipient typically feels centered and in touch with himself in a way that is very natural, but too rarely experienced by adults living a frantic postmodern lifestyle. The sense of well-being lingers, and people frequently report an immediate improvement in sleep.

Your actual experience of Reiki may center on physical, mental, or emotional changes—a sense of relaxation, relief from pain, greater clarity, a gradual lessening of

---

*Please note that the term *Reiki* refers both to primordial consciousness and to this practice we use to access primordial consciousness for healing and spiritual growth.

anxiety or expectations or other worrisome thoughts. Meanwhile, something far subtler is happening in the background. Very gently, very quietly, very gradually, Reiki opens an inner spiritual connection that can significantly change the way a person experiences life, a sense of connectedness that can help transform negative attitudes and create a sense of meaning and purpose. This may be the most valuable gift Reiki offers.

Of all the statements I've heard about Reiki's benefits, the most common—and the most profound—is simply "I feel better about myself." Feeling better about ourselves is the cornerstone of well-being. This shift begins with the first treatment and is strengthened by each successive session.

WHERE DID REIKI COME FROM?

Reiki as we know it today originated in the early twentieth century in Japan with a householder and lifelong spiritual aspirant named Mikao Usui. Drawing from years of experience and a profound revelation during a three-week fasting retreat, Usui organized a body of spiritual practices that included healing practices which he taught from 1922 until his death in 1926. Usui had an unusually expansive vision for his time and culture, and offered his beginning practices openly, teaching some two thousand Japanese students. From that point, students progressed to different levels depending upon their commitment to regular practice. Fewer than twenty senior students were trained to continue Usui's work. One of these students was a medical doctor retired from the navy named Chujiro Hayashi, who opened a clinic in Tokyo with Usui's blessing. Hawayo Takata, a first-generation Japanese-American, came to this clinic and became Hayashi's student after being relieved of her health problems. Hayashi and Takata collaborated to bring Reiki to America. Hayashi formally recognized Takata as a Reiki master in 1938. Takata continued to practice and teach in Hawaii, on the U.S. mainland, and in British Columbia, Canada, until her death in 1980. She left twenty-two students to continue her work. Reiki is now practiced around the world. (A more detailed overview of Reiki history is offered in chapter 3.)

DO I HAVE TO "BELIEVE" IN REIKI?

You need not *believe* in anything to benefit from Reiki. You only have to be open-minded enough to experience treatment. Religion involves adherence to a particular set of beliefs. Spirituality, on the other hand, is how each individual relates to the invisible parts of life, how we grapple with issues such as meaning and value. It is intensely personal and not optional. Although groups might have spiritual practices in common—meditation, contemplation, yoga, etc.—these practices are performed to develop each person's spiritual awareness, each person's individual relationship with the unseen, rather than in accordance with dogma. A person may be both religious and spiritual, or either one alone.

Reiki is not religious or dogmatic in any way. It developed, instead, out of a spiritual tradition, and sits at the intersection of science and spirit. Think of your first (few) Reiki treatments as an experiment. Observe the experience and note how you feel before and after. Although most people know very quickly if Reiki is of interest to them, for some the recognition takes longer. Give yourself the time you need.

HOW CAN REIKI HELP ME?

Reiki gently encourages a person's system toward its own unique balance. Because of this, Reiki can potentially benefit anyone, whether he or she is healthy and wants to stay that way or is addressing any kind of health concern. Artists use Reiki to expand creativity, and athletes find it speeds recovery. A teen calls it her mobile help plan and loves how fast Reiki works. Others appreciate how it strengthens intuition. The list of benefits is long and very personal, both because people are imbalanced in different ways and because they notice and value different changes.

Reiki may not be the only help you need, so it's important to know that Reiki combines well with interventions such as medications, surgery, acupuncture, chemotherapy, even psychotherapy. By enhancing your sense of well-being and helping your system regain balance, Reiki might even strengthen the benefits received from other health interventions. And there is no time when Reiki is dangerous. Even when physical cure is not possible, Reiki can still bring healing. This may show up as symptomatic relief from a chronic condition, feeling a willingness and even enthusiasm to take care of oneself (imagine actually wanting to exercise or quit smoking), or profound peacefulness at the time of death—a loved one's or even your own.

The stories of Jerry, Miguel and Carolyn are just a few examples of how Reiki can bring balance and create comfort for people facing health challenges. Not all stories of Reiki success are as clear-cut as theirs, of course; others receive from Reiki subtle enhancement or an overall feeling of calm permeating their everyday lives. People trained in Reiki can find relief simply by placing one or both of their Reiki hands (as we often refer to our hands after First Degree initiations) on themselves. In the midst of crisis, even a subtle improvement in well-being can be significant. People with chronic pain, for example, may aim to be painless, but they are grateful for any reduction in the intensity of their pain.

Carol, an accountant nearing fifty, came to me seeking relief from her migraines. Only later did I discover that she also suffered from panic attacks, hot flashes, and muscle spasms. In her mind, these were distinct and unrelated symptoms, and she could live with them. What she couldn't live with were the headaches.

After her first treatment, Carol expressed delight at how relaxed and renewed she felt. She was intrigued to hear she could learn Reiki, and promptly joined my next class. That was seven years ago. Although, like Miguel, many people using Reiki no longer suffer migraines, Carol's migraines didn't stop. Over time, however, they became less severe and occurred less frequently. Carol became more aware of subtle warning signs and discovered that giving herself even a brief Reiki treatment early in an attack would often subdue the headache. She also became aware of how hard driving she was and the effect that was having on her health.

Meanwhile, as she continued to receive Reiki, Carol became less anxious and felt more in control of her life. Not contemplative by nature, she turned to psychotherapy for self-discovery. Carol began exploring and letting go of anger and resentments she had previously retained as being justified. Her hot flashes all but disappeared, and her muscle spasms stopped. She continues to enjoy giving herself Reiki. With Reiki, it's not important to know how all Carol's symptoms were related other than that they were happening to the same person. And that's part of the beauty and ease of Reiki: We don't have to know.

There are two ways you can bring Reiki into your life. One is to receive treatment, either from a professional or from a friend who has been trained. The other option—and this is what makes Reiki unique—is to learn to practice Reiki yourself, so that you can give yourself a treatment whenever you like. I encourage all my clients, but especially those with serious illness or particularly stressful lifestyles, to learn Reiki self-care. Once you learn to practice, you can also share Reiki with your family, friends, and pets.

One of the best aspects of Reiki is that it can only help—it can never hurt. You cannot "overdose" on Reiki, no matter how many treatments you get or how long they last. Once you have taken what you need, Reiki hands become quiet and you receive only the simple comfort of caring touch. Ironically, the greatest challenge in Reiki can be appreciating how easy—and easeful—the process is. We are so used to working hard for what we want and need that we don't know how to just let life unfold.

It takes some time to recognize how deep the healing can go, and there is much that we will never know. We typically live so far away from a sense of well-being that we lose sight of what we are missing. But beyond the reduction in stress and pain, the steadying of mood, the expansion of self-awareness, the increased productivity, and more profound sense of engagement, lies the realm of prevention. We have no way of knowing what suffering we avoid by caring for ourselves regularly with Reiki. The symptomatic relief is the tip of the iceberg, the foundation of which is unseen, but may be felt. All this from the touch of a Reiki hand.

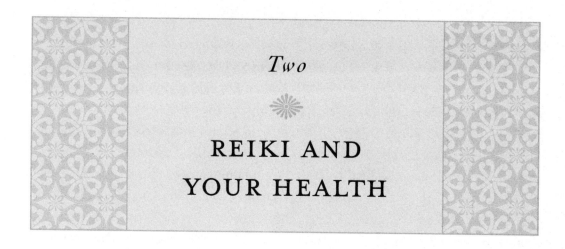

Two

REIKI AND YOUR HEALTH

If we don't change our course we will end where we are heading.

CHINESE PROVERB

Traditional, holistic medicine sees health as balance, a multileveled state of harmony and integrity both within the person (body/mind/spirit) and between the person and his environment (physical, social, and spiritual). Aware of the delicate complexity of these interrelationships, natural medicine seeks to strengthen the individual's innate ability to balance and heal; interventions are used to stimulate movement toward balance rather than to override natural functioning.*[1]

Although the concept of balance is known in conventional medicine, biomedicine has increasingly focused on the ailments of specific body parts and left it up to the

---

*Balance does not preclude the value of a fighting spirit when addressing disease, but fighting is done from a place of acceptance and self-worth, not anger.

body's self-regulatory mechanisms to restore homeostasis.*[2] Twenty years ago I never dreamed that the holistic paradigm of a balanced system, which made such intuitive sense to me, would ever make sense to biomedicine, but something is clearly shifting. It's not just that conventional medicine is realizing traditional healing therapies are useful; biomedicine is finding evidence that supports the holistic perspective. For example, emerging evidence suggests that underlying conditions, such as inflammation, play unexpected roles in disease, contrary to previously held assumptions. It is now known that people diagnosed with one chronic inflammatory condition are more likely than other people to develop another inflammatory condition. A recent study found people with ulcerative colitis (UC) or Crohn's disease are more prone to arthritis, asthma, bronchitis, psoriasis, multiple sclerosis (MS), kidney disease, and pericarditis, with arthritis and asthma being most common.[3] A separate study found that UC and Crohn's disease patients have a higher incidence of MS and two other serious nervous system disorders, demyelination and optic neuritis.[4] These links have long been understood in Asian medicine, which identifies underlying conditions that express themselves in a range of ways in different people.

A HEALING LIFESTYLE

There is so much in life that weakens our well-being, including the passage of time, but often the negative effects of an unhealthy lifestyle don't show for fifteen to twenty years. While we have well-being, it is wise to do what we can to strengthen and protect our health. Our lives are busy, so we need something we can do easily every day, even several times a day if we feel under the weather. If we have a chronic health condition, we need something we can do to relieve our symptoms and to encourage our overall sense of well-being. If we are confronting a life-threatening diagnosis, we need something we can do between our trips to the doctor, something that will restore

---

*Guyton and Hall's *Textbook of Medical Physiology* defines homeostasis as the "maintenance of static or constant conditions in the internal environment."

our sense of wholeness and our visceral memory of health. When we receive a serious diagnosis, we need healing on several fronts. We need to heal the illness. We need to heal the underlying condition leading to the illness, which has been building up for many years. We need to heal the trauma of the diagnosis. We need something that will make us more comfortable and help balance the side effects of medications and needed medical procedures. We also need to grow into a more healthful way of being with ourselves.

Michael Gnatt, M.D., sat opposite a patient who, in her seventies, still took dance class. Katherine had polyps and a family history of colon cancer. She had regular screenings, and was told she could wait five years before the next checkup. Three and a half years later, she followed her intuition that something was wrong and was diagnosed with colon cancer. Sitting with her internist, she was so agitated with grief, fear, and rage that she couldn't address important treatment decisions. Seeing that they were at an impasse, Gnatt invited her to the treatment table for Reiki. Twenty minutes later, Katherine was refreshed and centered. By the next day, she had sorted out exactly what treatment she wanted, and where. She said her Reiki treatment was like dancing, in that she felt her breath move throughout her body.

Reiki can provide quiet, steady support for all levels of healing and growth. For those who choose to learn to practice Reiki, that support is as always within reach. Just adding Reiki can transform our lifestyle into a healthful one. As a young woman with lupus said, "With the help of Reiki, I am able to choose new ways of being that have invited balance, harmony and wholeness into my life."

HEALTH BASICS

A very simple holistic perspective identifies three functions our bodies need to perform optimally in order to maintain health and well-being: We need to breathe well, sleep well, and digest well. When these functions are optimized, we feel good overall and we have resilience. We can think of stress as anything that compromises these functions. Any loss of well-being is accompanied by a loss of functioning in at least one of these three areas, which quickly spreads to the others. Such weakened functioning is often subclinical, below the radar of biomedicine, but nonetheless undermines health and well-being.

When breathing, sleep, or digestion is weakened, we need to intervene to regain and maintain balanced, healthy function in all three areas. Sometimes rest alone is sufficient, but in today's world, the art of resting has largely been lost. This is where Reiki can help. It gently carries you along the path to deep rest. As Reiki provides deep relaxation, the spiraling effects of stress begin to unravel. By improving breathing, sleep, and digestion, Reiki restores the functions that lead to recovery and wellness. Let's take a closer look at each of these vital functions.

Breathing

Healthy breathing is often overlooked, yet it is through the breath that tension and anxiety are naturally dissipated. When we breathe well, air is filtered and humidified by the nose, oxygen enters the bloodstream, carbon dioxide is exhaled, and inner organs receive gentle stimulation as the diaphragm expands and contracts and the ribs open.

Under stress, unhealthy breathing patterns such as mouth breathing and hyperventilation may occur, and stress can aggravate conditions such as asthma and chronic bronchitis. When we don't breathe well, we may suffer from congestion in the nose or chest, or even lack adequate oxygen, and accumulate carbon dioxide. Not breathing well affects our state of mind and our ability to sleep.

Reiki treatment precipitates a rapid response in breathing for practitioner and recipient alike. Breathing typically shifts even as treatment is just beginning, with the breath becoming freer, more rhythmic, and open. As treatment progresses and the recipient approaches a profound state of meditative relaxation, the breath may become very quiet, as happens in deep meditation. (Yoga texts speak in depth about the connection between the breath and one's mental state.)[5]

I was called to the ICU to treat a man of the cloth in his sixties, a vibrant community leader who had been hospitalized for a couple of weeks with an unclear diagnosis. It was painful for his wife of many years to see her husband restrained as he ranted in his bed. She knew nothing of Reiki but, desperate to effect a change in her husband's state, decided to follow a friend's recommendation. The minister was taking thirty or more breaths per minute when I began treatment (normal is twelve to sixteen). The monitor traced the change as he began to breathe more normally. By the end of the hour, he was breathing just slightly faster than normal and was no longer agitated. He was moved out of the ICU the next day.

Sleep

We all know the velvety texture of deep sleep. We awake clearheaded, with a sense of the sweetness of life. The body and mind experience a natural phase of detoxification and rejuvenation during deep sleep that is irreplaceable (except perhaps by profound meditation).

Difficulty sleeping is usually the first recognized symptom of stress, even though compromised breathing actually occurs first. If persistent, sleep disturbance or deprivation can lead to fatigue, difficulty concentrating, achy muscles (as occurs in fibromyalgia), and impaired immune functioning. Fatigue often leads to overeating and/or reliance on stimulants in a misguided attempt to restore vitality, both of which disrupt natural digestive rhythms and our ability to nourish ourselves.

People receiving Reiki often relax into a deep, sleeplike meditative state that is profoundly refreshing to body and mind. Whether or not this happens, even people with a long history of insomnia often sleep better the first night after Reiki treatment or their first Reiki class. Many of my Reiki students, particularly those who are HIV+, have had to take medications that interfered with sleep. Sleeping medications didn't solve the problem and left them groggy the next day. Students reported improved sleep once they began practicing Reiki on themselves, and many were able to stop taking sleeping medications altogether.

Sharon was a dynamic television producer whose career was cut short when she suffered damage to both sides of her brain after falling at work. Several years later, she still had constant pain, memory loss, and difficulty concentrating, and she walked with a cane. Sharon called her doctor when a new pain began in the right side of her neck and jaw. A few minutes of Reiki in his office gave her such relief that her doctor referred her to me for continued treatment. During our first session, Sharon was surprised that she dozed off a few times. She took a nap later that day and slept through the night for the first time in years. It occurred to her that the years of sleeplessness had contributed to her accident.

Digestion

It is through the capacity to digest that we are nourished. And it is not simply our food that is digested; we need also to digest our experiences.

When we make it a point to eat well, choosing fresh food appropriate to the season and the time of day, sitting down in a calm environment and taking time to chew, and sitting for a while afterward or taking a gentle stroll, the body is able to use the nutrients efficiently and, just as efficiently, eliminate the waste. When we don't attend to our digestive needs, the food we eat becomes toxic in our systems and the toxins gravitate toward the area of our constitutional weakness, setting the stage for disease.

Digestive upset may manifest as symptoms typical of irritable bowel syndrome, such as diarrhea, constipation, abdominal cramping, and nausea. Stress can aggravate chronic digestive diseases such as inflammatory bowel disease (ulcerative colitis and Crohn's disease).

The digestive tract's response to Reiki can be quite audible, with the abdominal gurgling called borborygmus frequently heard soon after the session starts. Clients often feel embarrassed and are quick to blame these noises on having had coffee, not having had coffee, just having finished a meal, having skipped a meal, or whatever is happening in their lives. I reassure them this belly music is a good thing, a clear sign that the body is responding and normalizing.

Digestive improvement shows up in many ways. Some people notice their appetite returns, or find themselves attracted to more healthful foods or enjoying preparing meals. Many experience a return to normal bowel function, even after a long history of constipation. Symptoms of irritable bowel syndrome or Crohn's disease may be calmed by a single session, but repeated treatment will give deeper balancing and longer-lasting benefits.

REIKI AND INSOMNIA

In 2004, I gave a presentation and taught Reiki at the Integrative Approaches to Depression conference sponsored by the Program in Integrative Medicine at the University of Arizona. I was riveted by the presentation given by Rubin Naiman, Ph.D., clinical assistant professor of medicine at the Program in Integrative Medicine and sleep specialist at Tucson's Miraval Resort. Naiman's lecture and our subsequent conversations gave me the scientific backstory for what I had long observed in my clients.

According to Naiman, it's rare to find Americans who are still experiencing deep sleep by their fiftieth birthday. He sees sleep disorders as the number-one health problem in the United States, and offers statistics to back that up. Sleep disorders such as insomnia, obstructive sleep apnea (OSA), restless leg syndrome (RLS), and period limb movement disorder (PLM) afflict well in excess of 100 million Americans, yet they remain underdiagnosed and undertreated. Eighty percent of psychiatric patients have sleep disorders, and the severity of insomnia correlates with intensity of symptoms. Insomnia, which affects approximately 60 million American adults, is a very common symptom of depression and also a risk factor for becoming depressed. In fact, one year of insomnia is the strongest predictor of subsequent clinical depression.

The broad consequences of sleep disorders are illustrated by the association of daytime sleepiness with eating, especially among women, and the fact that evening is the most common period of substance use. Naiman notes the overlapping symptoms of depression and sleepiness—social withdrawal, fatigue, and difficulty concentrating. In addition, he articulates reasons to find nonpharmacological remedies for sleep disturbances. Beyond the obvious fact that it is generally better to take less medication, Naiman points out that all sleep medications have unwanted side effects. Medications are relentless, he says, pushing the brain toward unconsciousness without giving the profound benefits of deep sleep. Newer sleeping pills like Ambien and, more recently, Lunesta tout benefits over older medications and appear to be safer. There are still significant problems with these drugs, however. Beyond resulting in dependence and habituation, we do not know their long-term effects. They can be associated with morning grogginess or cognitive deficit, and, most significant, they undermine our sense of self-efficacy around letting-go into sleep.

Although there has not yet been any research on Reiki and sleep, formerly sleepless Reiki students have reported Reiki helping in a number of ways. People who had trouble falling asleep find an early evening Reiki practice session helps them get back into their normal cycle of wakefulness and sleepiness. Reiki enables many adults to sleep through the night again. And when students awaken during the night, Reiki self-treatment keeps them from becoming anxious, so they can fall back to sleep.

People beginning Reiki treatment commonly report deeper, more refreshing sleep, whether they notice themselves sleeping more or less. Occasionally I hear reports of greater dream activity when first experiencing Reiki. Naiman says this can happen as people return to their natural sleep cycle.

Naiman sees rest as the secret ingredient in all healing approaches: "Rest is a low-grade form of sleep. The same neurochemical process underlies both rest and sleep. Although that process is biochemically complex, a simple explanation is that the brain slows down. You cannot sleep well unless you know how to rest." Reiki's role in creating better rest, then, is important.

If Reiki improves the ability to sleep, it may be activating the body's repair mechanisms and resetting the body's ability to self-regulate. This might explain why Reiki has been seen anecdotally to bring benefit in such a range of situations, including serious, often unresponsive conditions such as anorexia and bulimia. For conditions such as these, clearly Reiki is not the only treatment needed, but it can be useful as a continuing support, particularly for those who learn and practice Reiki self-treatment, and as a gateway to other needed therapies.

Eating disorders aside, the link between inadequate sleep and weight gain is well documented and may involve more than simply overeating. If you are carrying unwanted weight, even if it's the beginning of the slow creep of middle-aged pounds, read on.

REIKI AND WEIGHT MANAGEMENT

We all want weight management to be easy, but for many of us, it's not. Yes, there are some fortunate people who can eat a little less at each meal or step up their activity—or both—and drop five pounds in no time. Then there's the rest of us. Either we don't really make the effort, or we make what seems like reasonable effort without getting reasonable results. This is because excess weight is often more complicated than we think, and Reiki can help. If you are struggling with weight, take a deep breath and keep reading.

Some people lose weight after incorporating Reiki into their lifestyle. Georgia had hovered on the brink of quitting smoking for years, and registered for Reiki training hoping it would seal her resolve. Stopping at Starbuck's en route to her First Degree class, she surprised herself by ordering green tea instead of her usual venti latte. Over the next year, as Georgia practiced Reiki self-treatment daily, she slowly and effortlessly dropped thirty pounds of body weight and thirty points of blood pressure. She has not had a cup of coffee since that first green tea, and she still smokes, but less.

How might Reiki help with weight loss? There are probably a number of mechanisms involved, particularly when the weight loss is as effortless as Georgia's. It is likely that regular Reiki treatment is reducing the amount of stress hormones in the blood that incline the body to hold weight. Other possible reasons include improved overall digestive function, gradual detoxification, more refreshing sleep, enhanced hormonal balance, becoming more in tune with one's body, gravitating to what it truly needs, less emotional eating, feeling better overall, and feeling better about oneself. The better we feel, the more likely we will make the choices and the effort that improve well-being. Which means that Reiki can be the change that makes it easier for us to make other needed changes.

From a holistic perspective, weight gain is not itself a problem but rather a symptom of deeper, multifaceted dysfunction. Each person who *struggles* with excess weight has a unique imbalance and needs an individualized approach. This means finding a health-care professional who can identify what's happening (or not happening) in *your* body and create a concrete, individualized lifestyle plan for you (if it were any easier, you'd have had success already). You may not be able to find this kind of guidance within the strict confines of conventional medicine, which is, after all, standardized medicine and can't really address the needs of the outliers. Rather, this is a place where experienced practitioners of Asian medical systems—Ayurveda, Tibetan, or Chinese medicine—can be very helpful.

Rather than insist on standardized dietary recommendations, indigenous medical systems see food as medicine. Food is most nourishing when eaten within the context of the individual's constitution and current state of health, and appropriately to both time of day and season of the year. John Douillard explains the Ayurvedic approach to balanced eating clearly and in contemporary terms in *The Three Season Diet*. This book can help you recognize your body's unique needs in the moment so that you can make more informed food choices and consume foods in ways that support your health.

REIKI IS ALWAYS SAFE

Reiki treatment is safe in any situation. Reiki gently influences your individual system toward balance. Whether treatment comes from your own hands or someone else's, there is nothing invasive about how Reiki is administered. Reiki touch is light and not manipulative, so Reiki can be used even when people cannot be massaged. If there are burns or an open wound, the Reiki practitioner's hand can be held just above the body. Rather than being directed by the practitioner, Reiki activates according to the need of the person receiving the treatment, so there is no question of wrong dosage.

For these reasons, there are no known medical contraindications to using Reiki, no time when Reiki is dangerous. And Reiki can be valuable in any situation. Although people sometimes have amazing responses to Reiki treatment, you are wise to remember that Reiki may not be the only treatment needed; be sure to get all the care called for in your situation. When other care is required, it's good to know that Reiki combines safely with any conventional or complementary treatment.

Patients and care providers often observe how Reiki smooths the course of conventional treatment, perhaps enhancing its effectiveness. At the very least, a patient who is composed, one whose blood is not carrying a truckload of stress hormones, is less likely to have an adverse reaction to a test or treatment and more likely to receive optimal benefit.

Conventional medications and procedures tend to be unidirectional; they strongly move the person in one direction regardless of what else is happening in the person's system. Because of this, they frequently cause side effects. It's rather like knocking over a glass of water while you're rearranging the furniture to clear a walkway. Reiki helps with side effects because it restores harmony and cooperation in the body as much as possible at the time. Reiki takes the whole picture into account and since it does not have a set process of its own, Reiki embraces the strengthening aspects of the medical treatment and supports the body in addressing the treatment's unbalancing aspects. Reiki will never override the healing process of a conventional or complementary intervention. It will not, for example, undo the benefits of a medication or a medical procedure, but it will support recovery from the side effects.

The safety and value of Reiki and other complementary therapies in the treatment of even serious illnesses such as HIV and cancer are increasingly recognized in conventional medical centers. As Gary Deng, M.D., Ph.D., and Barrie R. Cassileth, Ph.D., of New York's Memorial Sloan-Kettering Cancer Center, one of the top cancer hospitals in the world, wrote:

> The judicious integration of touch therapies, mind-body therapies, acupuncture, and other complementary therapies into cancer patient care is warranted. Given patient interest, these therapies are likely to reduce troubling physical and emotional symptoms, offer patients a measure of control over their well-being, enhance quality of life, and improve both patient satisfaction and the physician-patient relationship.[6]

REIKI AND CHRONIC ILLNESS

People often ask me if I have treated a particular condition that they or their children have, such as cancer, or MS, or cystic fibrosis, or arthritis—the list is long. I always respond that Reiki doesn't treat disease; Reiki helps restore balance. And being balanced helps maintain normal functioning. As adults, we're often at the extreme states, confusing exhaustion with relaxation and caffeination with alertness. After Reiki treatment, we remember how we felt as kids, centered in ourselves, with enough energy to do what we wanted without feeling stressed, anxious, or tense. Of course, such a shift in our state is welcome at any time, but it can be particularly dramatic to those who are addressing chronic illness, with the additional anxiety and the feeling of being overwhelmed that illness brings, as well as side effects of medications. The empowerment of learning Reiki self-treatment eases the frustration associated with chronic disease.

If you think of Reiki as an effective destressor (and chapter 13 discusses research that supports this perspective), the benefits Reiki offers are the same benefits as removing stress from your body and your life. While there is as yet no research evidence that Reiki can slow the progression of chronic disease, there is some evidence that Reiki lowers stress hormones, and stress hormones hasten disease progression.

Reiki enhances well-being in ways that go beyond mere stress reduction, including emotional resolution, a sense of peace and acceptance, and increased self-awareness that lead to making more healthful choices. These changes help people turn their encounter with disease into a transformative process. They connect with parts of themselves that have remained hidden or underutilized, open new avenues for support, and find inner resources that further empower their healing.[7] One lupus patient said she learned Reiki self-treatment in the hope of reducing her medications (which she was able to do), but what she didn't expect was how strongly Reiki practice centered her in herself, enabling her to make profound, healthful shifts in her family relationships. She said, "It was the one thing that could connect me to myself and touch all of the pain and rage I was holding and it healed me."

The shift in well-being precipitated by Reiki treatment helps motivate people to create a more healthful lifestyle, as is necessary for dealing well with chronic conditions such as Type 2 diabetes. Although a serious disease, Type 2 diabetes usually causes only mild or no symptoms, making it easier for diabetics to be in denial about being at increased risk of nerve dysfunction, kidney and eye disease, and heart attacks, and to forget that the choices they make every day will significantly affect their future well-being. The beneficial effect of Reiki on diabetes control I have observed with many people I have treated or trained (including lower glucose and reduced dose of insulin) may be in part a result of helping them shift to a healthier lifestyle. Also, as Reiki reduces stress hormones, including cortisol and adrenaline, diabetes control would be expected to improve.

The following reflects my clinical experience and holistic perspective. As you read, please keep two things in mind: First, you are an individual, not a statistic, and your healing experience is unique. Second, all of the benefits we see with Reiki are the by-products of restoring balance from a very deep, subtle level. Some people respond faster and more dramatically than others. Some are more aware of what's happening than are others. Some people don't notice particular changes at first, but they just feel better overall, more optimistic, less stressed, less sad or angry or withdrawn.

Reiki and Nervous-System Disorders and Hormonal Imbalances

Hormonal imbalances and neurological conditions typically respond quickly to Reiki treatment. Since the nervous and endocrine systems regulate functions throughout the body, maintaining natural rhythms and organizing the staggeringly complex levels of self-regulation and repair that maintain health, it seems likely that the responsiveness of these systems to Reiki is a large part of how Reiki can benefit people with a wide range of conditions (it is also possible that the endocrine-system response is mediated through the nervous system).

Even people with long-standing imbalances can benefit from Reiki treatment. Reiki can be particularly helpful addressing the uncertainty that comes with a diagnosis of MS. Alzheimer's patients are often calmed by Reiki treatment, and people with Parkinson's disease may find relief from tremors, muscle tension, and agitation. Reiki can soothe painful neuropathy caused by disease or medication. The mother of one of my students who also had a teenage son with cerebral palsy approached me to teach them both to practice Reiki. In the years since, she has found that Reiki calms her son even when he is in the hospital for tests or surgery (which makes him very anxious) and seems to lessen the occurrence and intensity of spasms. Reiki also can be helpful with epilepsy or undiagnosed seizure disorders.

Reiki is safe in pregnancy and childbirth and while breast-feeding infants. It can also be useful in treating infertility and miscarriages. Women's menstrual cycles usually normalize or at least improve with the first cycle and often during the week of First Degree class. One student who had a self-described twenty-five-year history of "premenstrual rage" experienced no PMS during her next cycle. Others have found Reiki helpful with endometriosis, ovarian cysts, fibroids, and polycystic breasts.

Reiki and Inflammatory Conditions

Inflammation occurs in response to injury or infection as part of the normal healing process. In inflammatory diseases such as arthritis, the body's ability to regulate inflammation has been lost. The balance brought by Reiki treatment can be valuable in preventing or minimizing flare-ups. People with arthritis who receive Reiki treatment often report lessening of pain and increased mobility.

Reiki and Autoimmune Conditions

Ayurveda, the indigenous medical system of the subcontinent of India, speaks of the loss of access to the body's natural wisdom that accompanies the onset and progression of disease. This is never more obvious than in autoimmune conditions, when the body loses the ability to distinguish "self" from "intruder" and literally attacks itself. As an infusion of consciousness, does Reiki help reconnect the body with its innate wisdom? We can only theorize.

Practicing Reiki self-treatment may be particularly poignant for people with autoimmune diseases, empowering them to self-balance even as their bodies are engaged in self-attack. As one of my students with lupus wrote, "One of the most amazing aspects of my Reiki practice, which has been very healing, is having the power to take care of myself at any moment. And that has healed something on a deep level."

Reiki and Cardiac Disease

Holistic medicine links the heart with the emotions and with spirit, and there is emerging research evidence to support this. For example, research suggests that anger can trigger a fatal arrhythmia or stroke in people at high risk.[8] Other studies show that patients who have had heart attacks and are depressed are twice as likely to die or have a repeat attack.[9]

People report feeling more centered and emotionally balanced, more able to let go of past hurts and resentments, once they start using Reiki. Not only is a lessening of depression commonly reported by Reiki students, but also there are research data suggesting Reiki can have a lasting benefit for people with depression (discussed in chapter 13). In the first days after the shock of an emergency cardiac procedure, one longtime Reiki practitioner found that lying with his hands on his chest eased him through the emotional and physical trauma. It softened the grip of anxiety, enabling him to deeply rest and sleep peacefully in spite of the severity of his medical situation. A new client decided to learn to practice Reiki when her blood pressure dropped a healthy thirty-five points after her first treatment.

Reiki and Cancer

Reiki is used by cancer patients for relief from the anxiety, pain, and fatigue that can accompany every stage of the illness and treatment, and to support recovery beyond the active treatment phase.[10] For example, Reiki can reduce the relentless anxiety that stalks people awaiting diagnosis without interfering with the diagnostic process. After diagnosis, Reiki centers patients, enabling them to address treatment decisions with greater clarity. Reiki can help with side effects of treatment such as nausea and fatigue. And Reiki is an invaluable support after treatment, when patients often feel abandoned once they are cut loose from their treatment schedule to dwell alone in a land between illness and wellness. You may want to read my paper "Reiki for Mind, Body, and Spirit Support of Cancer Patients," published in the peer-reviewed medical journal *Advances in Mind-Body Medicine* 22(2) (Fall 2007) and bring it to your oncologist. It can be downloaded at http://www.advancesjournal.com/adv/web_pdfs/miles.pdf.

Reiki and Infectious Disease

Since Reiki is balancing, it can reduce susceptibility to infections, speed recovery from acute infections, and be a valuable part of the comprehensive treatment of HIV and other chronic infectious disease. Research is beginning to link Reiki with enhanced immune function (see chapter 13), which may be tied to Reiki's ability to soothe digestion (much of the immune system is in the gut). Improved digestion also makes it easier to get the nourishment needed to maintain strength. And Reiki helps balance the side effects of medications used to treat HIV, including antivirals.

Reiki and Mental Illness

Reiki's balancing effect can be valuable to people with a wide range of mental illnesses, and, depending on the severity of the symptoms, may enable them to reduce or even stop medications, with the supervision of their physicians. Since it is very common for people to need less medication once they include Reiki in their care, I encourage you to share your Reiki experience with your psychiatrist (you may want to read chapter 11). People who choose to learn to practice Reiki self-treatment seem to benefit from the empowerment of being able to address symptoms as they arise. A bipolar student wrote to me about how Reiki has helped him retain balance through a period of turbulent circumstances. He also remarked that Reiki is the first thing he's ever felt motivated to practice on a daily basis for any length of time.

Reiki in the Waiting Room

Anyone with chronic illness spends more time than she would like in waiting rooms. If you are a Reiki student, let Reiki help you with your medical visits. Consultations and tests, especially if done at clinics, usually involve considerable waiting. Bring something to read, bring a notebook for journaling (and taking notes during the consultation), but also use this time for Reiki. You may feel too conspicuous going through all the hand placements, but you can discreetly place a hand or hands on your abdomen, midriff, possibly even at your heart. Placing your hands atop your head may be both physically and psychologically uncomfortable, but if you lean forward and place your head in your hands, people are likely to just think you have a headache.

EMERGENCY REIKI

Reiki can also safely be used in any emergency. You can offer a patient Reiki with one hand while dialing 911 with the other. Even moments of Reiki can calm and stabilize a patient, thereby facilitating emergency medical interventions. If you are able to place your hand on the crown or over the solar plexus or heart, do so, but know that since the patient activates Reiki as needed, even one hand anywhere on the body can make a difference. Reiki can also be offered through a cast. In the case of burns or an open wound, hold your hand just above the injured area. The use of Reiki in emergency medicine is discussed in chapter 11.

REIKI AND SURGERY

If you are having surgery, you may want to use Reiki to support you before, after, or possibly during the operation. Recent studies have shown that even necessary surgery can have unanticipated and far-ranging repercussions. In addition to the risk of the surgical procedure, general anesthesia carries risk. Patients scheduled for ambulatory surgery are more likely to require admission to the hospital if the surgery lasts longer than sixty minutes.[11] The longer the time spent under general anesthesia, the greater the risk of dying during the first year after surgery.[12] Although the studies looked at noncardiac surgeries, most deaths were caused by heart attacks or cancer. Noncardiac surgery is also related to a cognitive decline in seniors up to two years later. Researchers theorize that the body responds to the stress of surgery with an inflammatory response that takes a long time to become balanced, if at all. Reiki can be used to help people with anxiety before surgery and also to rebalance the body afterward.

Mehmet Oz, M.D., renowned cardiac surgeon on staff at Columbia-Presbyterian Medical Center in New York City and coauthor of *You, The Owner's Manual: An Insider's Guide to the Body That Will Make You Healthier and Younger,* refers to surgery as "controlled trauma." Every day he performs lifesaving, traumatizing surgeries. Oz appreciates that healing comes from more than conventional medical know-how. He is committed to providing his patients with what they want to support their well-being. I have been fortunate to work with some of his patients who requested Reiki, offering it before, during, and after their open-heart surgery.

Oz does not experience a Reiki practitioner in the operating room as an intrusion. He says his patients attribute a sense of comfort and safety to Reiki, but notes that the benefits are subjective and difficult to measure. There have not yet been any studies looking at Reiki's effect on length of hospital stay, infection, or use of pain medication—areas ripe for research.

Unless I am actually in the operating room during surgery, my clients' surgeons don't know their patients are receiving Reiki. But surgeons have a clear appreciation of where their work ends and the body's healing mechanisms take over. They have performed their surgeries countless times and know the recovery curve. When a patient recovers faster than usual, surgeons notice.

Patients who have received Reiki delight in repeating their surgeons' astonished comments upon visiting them the next morning. I frequently hear physicians or nurses remark that the patient is recovering three times faster than the norm. Just a couple of hours after her patient's valve replacement surgery, one bemused ICU nurse told me he was really too healthy to be there. "Do me a favor," I said, smiling, "and keep him anyway."

COMBINING REIKI WITH OTHER COMPLEMENTARY THERAPIES

Reiki combines equally well with other complementary or traditional medical interventions. Patients who access complementary therapies outside medical settings are often proactive in their health care and appreciate the empowerment of learning Reiki self-treatment. Reiki students often place hands on themselves while receiving other treatment, sensing that Reiki's harmonizing influence makes them more receptive to healing and balances the session.

Subtle Therapies

Reiki mixes well with acupuncture, shiatsu, acupressure, and all forms of energy medicine, including marma therapy (Ayurvedic touch therapy). Remember that Reiki is balancing and does not have a treatment pathway of its own. Acupuncturists, shiatsu practitioners, and other subtle energy healers are sometimes mistakenly concerned that Reiki might bring too much energy into the patient's system and interfere with their treatment (I've only heard this question come up when receiving treatment from others, not regarding self-treatment). If you remember that Reiki activates only according to the need of the recipient, you can assuage any concerns. Explain that your Reiki practitioner is not directing Reiki into you but is merely a conduit through which healing vibrations flow as needed. If your practitioner remains unconvinced, you might agree not to have a Reiki treatment on the same day as your other treatment—not because this is necessary, but simply to accommodate your practitioner.

However, many acupuncturists and shiatsu therapists are Reiki trained and use Reiki during their sessions to align with the client and give a smoother, more effective treatment. Chinese practitioners have commented to me on Reiki's ability to heal meridians that have been cut in surgery. Although the physical tissues usually heal on their own, we can't assume the subtle channels will reconnect on their own. The disruption in the flow of chi through the meridians can damage health in unexpected ways. Without proper flow of chi, the organs are not nourished optimally. This may be an underlying factor in the increased incidence of medical problems in the year after surgery. Reiki helps restore these subtle pathways and balance the body from the stress of surgery.

Homeopathy

Classical homeopathy is really a form of energy medicine, even though it uses ingested remedies. Each remedy carries the vibrational essence of the source from which the remedy is derived, and the vibrations are what precipitate healing. I have used classical homeopathy since the mid-1970s, and it is one of my favorite healing modalities. Homeopathy can be very effective when used by a skilled practitioner, bringing fast results in acute situations and creating profound healing when used constitutionally for chronic conditions. Yet homeopathy is notoriously sensitive to interference. For this reason, and to avoid suppressing symptoms, homeopaths generally prefer their patients not to mix modalities. That said, homeopaths have referred patients to me for Reiki to soothe the discomfort of a strenuous healing crisis (a temporary, curative worsening of symptoms). Since Reiki supports the individual's unique balance and has no pathways of its own, Reiki treatment eases the patient through the crisis, allowing the imbalance to move more gracefully out of the system. I have seen patients come through a healing crisis with Reiki and move gently and quickly into the next stage of treatment.

Another time when Reiki can be useful to homeopathic treatment is when it is unclear which remedy is timely. Homeopaths often elect simply to wait until things sort themselves out, but a single Reiki treatment can safely and naturally speed that process. This is also true of conventional medicine. Since Reiki influences the system toward balance, Reiki treatment can help clarify the picture and facilitate medical diagnosis.

Meditation and Yoga

Reiki is a natural adjunct to meditation in that both these practices have the same goal, connecting with the inner source of stillness and peace. Students who are already meditating regularly when they learn Reiki report their meditation practice becoming more easeful, deeper, more pleasurable. Those who have previously found it difficult to meditate have expressed how gently Reiki opened that inner space to them.

The various practices of yoga, especially meditation, breathing techniques, postures, and self-study, have been part of my life since I was an adolescent. Both hatha yoga (the practice of physical postures, or *asanas*) and Reiki are spiritual healing practices that arose from meditation experiences and that normalize flow throughout the biofield (and thus the body). Practicing asanas, however, is as physically active as Reiki is physically passive. Asana practice grounds the subtle experience of Reiki in the physical body while Reiki increases our awareness of the subtle changes that happen during asana practice, *and* of the body's wisdom guiding us into alignment. Those who practice yoga athletically, like athletes of other sports, find that Reiki supports recovery from intense physical effort.

As discussed, good breathing, varying according to the need of the moment, is vital for good health. Reiki treatment quickly precipitates a shift toward more relaxed, healthful breathing. You may want to explore the natural link between Reiki (as both consciousness and practice) and the breath through the practice of *pranayama,* yogic breath control. If you are going to do anything more than simply relaxing into the natural breath—which for most of us is a lot— find a good teacher.* Reiki can bring you into a profound friendship with your breath, making you more aware of its subtleties.

---

*It is essential to find an experienced teacher who can teach pranayama practice safely and correctly. The following are good places to look for referrals in your area: www.anusara.com, www.kym.org, www.bksiyengaryoga.com.

This is definitely a practice in which less is more. For those who practice regularly, any combination of Reiki, meditation, postures, and pranayama gives a complete, practical experience of the omnipresence of consciousness, how it permeates every nook and cranny of our physical and subtle being.

Herbal Medicine

Reiki can be used simultaneously with herbal medicine. However, if you are taking herbs and having a healing crisis, don't rely on Reiki alone. Check with your herbalist, who may want to adjust the dosage or rethink the strategy.

Psychotherapy

Reiki practice and treatment enhance self-awareness, which is a great boon to any form of psychotherapy. It also creates a sense of inner safety that can be supportive when delving into difficult emotions and reevaluating painful memories. Many of my students have commented that their psychotherapy became more productive after they started receiving or practicing Reiki, regardless of the approach used. Reiki has a particular affinity with family therapy. Even if you are unable to work with a family therapist, you may find much to contemplate in the writings of Salvador Minuchin, M.D., one of the pioneers in the field.

Reiki, Healing, and Spiritual Engagement

Although Reiki treatment typically brings an immediate sense of relaxed, mindful well-being, the repercussions of Reiki as a spiritual healing practice are subtle and far-reaching. Like air or water, Reiki has no form of its own, and easily moves into forgotten crevices of our being bringing support and increasing awareness. Part of Reiki's healthful influence may be that the enhanced sense of well-being it brings inclines us toward other behaviors shown to be linked to good health. Feeling better makes it more likely that we will eat better; exercise; get adequate sleep; express our emotions honestly, clearly, and without undue rancor; maintain supportive social connections; and have the optimism that creates resilience.

Improving one's health often means making some changes. Self-efficacy is the recognition that we can make changes successfully. People who lack a sense of self-efficacy are less likely to make the changes needed. Enhanced well-being strengthens self-efficacy. Reiki can be the easy change that makes it possible to take creative ownership of one's life and make other needed changes.

People are more likely to heal if they are spiritually engaged. Many people, even those who consider themselves religious, don't have the tools to engage spiritually. Reiki can be a great asset here because it is a practice that has one foot in healing and one foot in spirituality. Reiki is a spiritual healing practice that has no dogma, no belief system. It gives people a simple practice to use at any time of the day or night, according to their lifestyle and preference.

Healing Retreats

No matter what your state of health, an intensive healing retreat is a powerful way to strengthen your well-being. Sequester yourself for a period of time, either in your home or elsewhere, so that you have nothing to do but focus on yourself and your inner life. A retreat is most powerful when there is absolutely no communication with the outside. That means no phone, no entertainment or distractions, not even music unless it is being used for sound healing. Arrange to have food available to you without intrusion.

Challenge yourself to express yourself in new ways in which you have no skill to hide behind. For example, if you are a visual artist, try drumming; if you are a musician, use crayons instead of your instrument.

You can benefit deeply from a solo retreat that includes ample Reiki self-treatment, silence, self-expression, and contemplation, or you can arrange to have other practitioners come to give silent treatments each day, even several times a day. If you are having practitioners come to give Reiki or other treatment, have someone else supervise the schedule so you are not distracted by the logistics. Especially if you have a serious illness, you will want to have a medical professional as part of the team or at least on backup.

Retreats are both a healing and an educational endeavor. When I organize a healing retreat for a client, I always include the learning of skills such as Reiki, meditation, yoga, ceremony, visualization, and journal-writing that the person in retreat can use to create a healing lifestyle after the retreat ends.

My students have supported each other during crisis by organizing themselves to offer daily hands-on treatment for three weeks, and by coordinating distant treatment.

Keeping Track

If you want to track Reiki's benefit to your well-being, list the symptoms that bother you the most, including stress and characteristics of which you are critical. When you have completed your list, review it and choose a few entries that you would like to track. It's easy to draw or compose on a computer a self-report survey called a visual analog scale (VAS) (see pages 216–17). Draw a horizontal line. At the left end, write 0 and "Not at all." At the right end, write 10 and "The worst I can imagine." Make a VAS for each entry that you want to track, and then make copies. To use the VAS, either mark an X at a place on the line that corresponds to your experience, or assign a number between 0 and 10 that describes it.

Here are two ways you might use your VAS sheets: You might fill one out before and one after each Reiki treatment you receive (either from yourself or someone else). Don't look back at the ratings on your before sheet until after you have completed the after sheet.

The other way to use your VAS sheets is to choose a time of day that suits you— perhaps before breakfast or at bedtime, or when you usually feel the worst—and fill out your self-survey at that time every day. If you have learned Reiki and are self-treating, gather your surveys for at least a week or so before comparing them. If you are receiving treatment from someone else, decide beforehand how long you will fill out your daily surveys before comparing them. Realize that there are always ups and downs. If you are using Reiki treatment over a period of time, you can average your scores for a week and see whether the averages improve over a period of at least a month. Because suffering is subjective, this kind of tracking can help you identify and appreciate the benefits Reiki treatment brings you.

It's never too late to incorporate Reiki into your well-being program. Regardless of whether you are thriving and want to stay that way, or you are in the throes of diagnostic tests, or are facing a serious health challenge, Reiki can help. As Michael Gnatt, M.D., says, "Reiki provides instant transformation out of the usual patterns of disregulation. Reiki puts you back in a healing mode."

Three

✳

THE STORY
OF REIKI

*My Usui Reiki Ryoho is original, never before explored,
and incomparable in the world.*

MIKAO USUI

In the communities that grow around practices such as Reiki or meditation or yoga, we refer to the lineage of our teachers. It's the ancestry of our practice, our family tree. It is the basis for our understanding of our practice. It honors those who have taught us, as well as the practice those teachers have imparted. The vast majority of people practicing Reiki in the world today share the same root lineage. Everyone practicing Reiki can thank the undisputed originator of this practice, Mikao Usui.

While one need not know the history of Reiki in order to practice, students are often curious about the origin of Reiki and how Reiki practice became available to people around the world.

The three people who made it possible for us to benefit from this simple, transformative practice lived in a world very different from ours. Each one overcame significant obstacles in order to carry the practice into the present with commitment and integrity.

MIKAO USUI

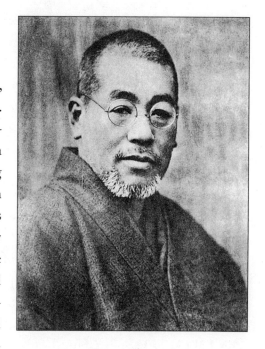

Mikao Usui
Courtesy Phyllis Lei Furumoto

The story of Reiki starts with Mikao Usui, who lived in Japan between 1865 and 1926. Usui was a spiritual seeker who was married and had two children, a son and a daughter.* Usui was a man of imposing physique and ready smile who persevered in the face of many obstacles. Although he was talented and capable, he encountered many setbacks as he tried to make his way in the world. Of a generally even and contented temperament, Usui was decisive in addressing challenges. He had wide interests and was an avid reader, educating himself in history, medicine, healing practices, and various spiritual philosophies and practices.

In his later years (perhaps in the spring of 1922), Usui went to Mount Kurama, a sacred site in Japan, for a long fasting retreat. Such a practice was not uncommon among serious spiritual aspirants. During the retreat, Usui had a profound meditation in which he sensed subtle vibrations above his head. Usui came to understand this experience as having awakened in him the power to heal, and to empower others to heal. After using this ability successfully on himself and his family, Usui decided to share it publicly and relocated his home to facilitate doing so.

---

*Most of what is known about Usui's life comes from the memorial erected by his students at the Saihoji Temple in Tokyo in 1927. The memorial text expresses the respect and gratitude Usui's students felt for him and gives us a glimpse into his life. Written as it was by students honoring their teacher after his death, we cannot assume it is precisely factual, but it paints a picture that helps us understand the roots of the practice known today as Reiki.

Usui's decision to share his gift publicly was a significant departure from Japanese custom, which was to share such treasures only with one's immediate circle. Usui gave more than two thousand Japanese students initiation, or *Reiju,* into First Degree Reiki practice, called *Shoden,* or basic teachings. Students were encouraged to continue attending group meetings with him.[1] Usui received many requests to travel and teach, and continued to do so until the end of his life. He died of a stroke in Fukuyama, the last stop on a trip that included Kure, Hiroshima, and Saga, at the age of sixty.

Usui's students credit their teacher's discipline and vast experience as the foundation that made it possible for him to create the practice of Reiki. Although characterized as an affable teacher, Usui did not suffer fools lightly. He could be impatient with students who didn't practice. The purpose of learning Reiki was to practice it in daily life. Usui specified that Reiki be taught simply, so that the practice could be easily understood and accessible to the wider public.

Usui referred to his practice as the "Secret of Happiness" and the "Secret of Medicine." This linking of happiness and healing is typical in Asian medicine, which understands spiritual well-being as the foundation of health. Usui's teachings were meant to improve body and mind, with *mind* including all nonphysical aspects of human life, mental, emotional, and spiritual. Usui's practice included recitation of Reiki Precepts.

In some Western Reiki circles today, there is argument about whether Usui's original practice was a spiritual practice or a healing practice. This is an argument that only Westerners could have. Asian culture does not make such distinctions. It can be said that Usui's practice focused on spiritual development with healing as a by-product, whereas Reiki, as it is often practiced today, tends to focus on healing with spiritual development as the by-product.

CHUJIRO HAYASHI

Among the twenty-one students whom Usui trained as Reiki masters[2] was a retired naval captain and medical doctor named Chujiro Hayashi (1878–1940). He began

studying with Usui in 1925. They collaborated on a handbook, which specified different hand placements for the treatment of
various conditions.

Usui's partnership with Hayashi in this
handbook implies a level of recognition from
the Reiki master for his student. Was this
gesture of distinction drawn by the enthusiasm and commitment Hayashi brought to
his practice? Was it because Hayashi was
Usui's only student who was also a medical
doctor? Usui had suffered two strokes a
year or so before the one that killed him.
Was he feeling his mortality and on the
alert for a student who shared his vision,
someone who might carry Reiki to the world
beyond his immediate sphere? We don't
know the answers to these questions. Usui

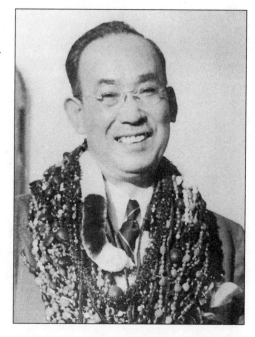

Chujiro Hayashi
Courtesy of Phyllis Lei Furumoto

encouraged Hayashi to open a clinic and develop the healing aspects of Reiki practice.

The passing of a teacher such as Usui leaves a complicated situation among the
remaining students, all wanting to honor their teacher but each having his own understanding about the direction Reiki should go in the future. When Usui died unexpectedly in 1926, Hayashi joined his fellow students in the Usui Reiki Ryoho Gakkai (Gakkai)
(Usui Reiki Healing Method Association), an organization that still exists in Japan today. Five or six years later, Hayashi left the Gakkai to start his own organization,
Hayashi Reiki Kenkyu Kai (Hayashi Reiki Research Association, or Hayashi Reiki
Study Group).

Around the same time, Hayashi further simplified the practice of Reiki, bringing it
closer to the way it would soon be introduced to the West. In Hayashi's clinic, people
received treatment from two practitioners simultaneously while lying on treatment
tables instead of sitting on tatami mats on the floor.

Even after starting his own organization, Hayashi taught and gave treatment in front of a scroll of Usui's Precepts. According to his student Chiyoko Yamaguchi (as told to her student Hyakuten Inamoto), Hayashi referred to his training as Usui Reiki Ryoho (Usui Reiki Treatment). Although neither Usui nor Hayashi was secretive about the practice, neither of them advertised.

HAWAYO TAKATA

The third important figure in the story of Reiki is a woman named Hawayo Takata. Takata was born at dawn on December 24, 1900, on the Hawaiian island of Kauai. Coming into the world just as the sun was rising over the mountains, Takata was named after the newly formed Territory of Hawaii, where her parents had emigrated

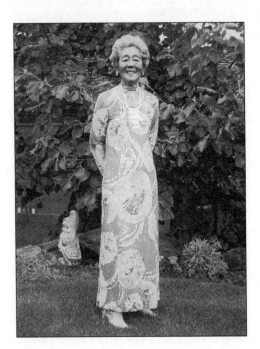

Hawayo Takata
Courtesy Phyllis Lei Furumoto

from Japan.[3] Her father worked on a sugarcane plantation, and Takata's early years were full of the hard work often seen in the lives of immigrants.

Takata married and had two daughters, but her husband died in 1930, leaving the young widow struggling to support her family. Her health broke under the strain. She needed surgery to remove gallstones as well as an abdominal tumor, but her asthma was too severe for her to tolerate anesthesia.[4] Then one of her sisters died suddenly while Takata's parents were spending a year in Japan. Rather than sending such a heartbreaking announcement by letter, Takata made her way to Japan, her two young daughters and sister-in-law in tow, to deliver the sad news in person.[5]

While in Japan, Takata sought medical treatment for her ailments. Her efforts to regain her health led her to the Reiki clinic of Chujiro Hayashi in Tokyo. She was escorted to a room with eight treatment tables, where sixteen male practitioners offered Reiki in pairs. Although Takata did not understand exactly what was being done as she lay fully clothed on the treatment table, she felt warmth and vibrations coming from the practitioners' hands. She listened as the practitioners made comments to each other about her ailments, and wondered how they could so accurately read the problems in her body.

Three weeks of daily Reiki treatments brought significant improvement to her health. Within four months of arriving at the clinic, Takata's health was restored.

Takata was loath to return to her difficult life in Hawaii and leave Reiki behind in Japan. She knew it would be just a matter of time before her health collapsed again. She was determined to be accepted as Hayashi's student. At this time, while Reiki was meant to be accessible, it was still considered uniquely Japanese, not to be shared outside the culture. Japanese protocol precluded Takata from making her request directly to Hayashi. How could a foreigner hope to be entrusted with this spiritual healing practice without showing respect for its culture of origin? Takata appealed to Dr. T. Maeda, a respected surgeon she knew also to be a friend of Hayashi.[6] Although initially reluctant to support such a radical request, he finally acquiesced. The surgeon composed a handwritten letter to Hayashi, expressing Takata's request. Hayashi was impressed and presented the matter to the directors of the Hayashi Reiki Kenkyu Kai for consideration.

Hayashi accepted Takata as his student on the provision that she study as all his students did: training and working in the clinic in the mornings and making afternoon house calls to patients too ill to travel. The Hayashis invited Takata to live in their house during this time. Takata offered to sell her house in Hawaii to finance her training.[7]

Takata's training was intensive: clinic in the morning, house calls in the afternoon, and a review of her day's work with Hayashi at dinner. Her understanding of and reliance on Reiki deepened, and her relationship to Reiki evolved as she came to understand that Reiki is more than healing vibrations in the hands.

Takata returned to Hawaii in the summer of 1937, and Hayashi and his daughter followed in September. They spent six months in Hawaii helping Takata introduce

Reiki to the territory, starting in Honolulu. Hayashi and Takata offered free lectures and demonstrations and received attention from the local Japanese newspaper. Takata assisted as Hayashi taught Reiki classes. When he left Hawaii in February of 1938, Hayashi announced that Takata was a fully accredited Reiki master, the only one outside of Japan.

Even though Hayashi had spent only a year with his Reiki master, Usui, and had been practicing Reiki for only fifteen years, his practice had profoundly changed him. Hayashi trained seventeen Reiki masters before he died on May 10, 1940. According to Takata, Hayashi foresaw World War II. A retired naval officer, he knew he would be conscripted to fight. Takata said Hayashi chose to die rather than be responsible for killing others. She said Hayashi died in meditation, as very advanced spiritual pactitioners are known to do. (It is also possible that Hayashi committed ritual suicide, which in Japanese culture at the time would have been an honorable way for him to avoid fighting.)

Takata continued practicing and teaching Reiki, primarily in Hawaii. Hayashi had warned Takata to stay away from the Japanese community during those troubled times, so she moved to a Filipino community, assuming Americans wouldn't be able to tell the difference. This is how she avoided unwanted attention from the authorities.[8] Even after the war ended, Japanese were not favored by Americans.

Takata moved to Honolulu, where she was based for nearly three decades, making occasional trips to the U.S. mainland. In the autumn of 1973, she was invited to teach in British Columbia. This began the final chapter of her life, in which the demand for classes eclipsed her clinical work. Teaching monopolized her last seven years.

In 1976, as the need for more teachers became apparent, and perhaps as she faced her own mortality, Takata began initiating students as Reiki masters. She had initiated only one master sometime earlier, her sister Kay Yamashita in Hawaii. Why Takata initiated her sister at that time is not known. Part of her motivation may have been to ensure that Reiki would continue in the West even if something happened to her.

Takata told one of her Canadian master students, Wanja Twan, that Hayashi had said Reiki would spread around the world and that people would change Reiki once it was brought out of Japan. Takata had reassured Hayashi, saying she would never change the practice, but clearly she wasn't seeing then what he was able to foresee.[9]

After attending many classes in British Columbia and listening to tapes of classes Takata had given in California, Twan noticed that Takata taught a bit differently in the United States from the way she did in Canada. The substance was the same, and the practice was the same, but Takata seemed aware of the cultural differences between the students in the two countries and was adept at speaking specifically to the people in front of her at any given time. The contrast between her experience of Takata in the mountains and the tapes of the California classes deeply impressed Twan. It reinforced her direct observation that Takata was in no way formulaic in her teaching. Rather, Takata was centered and pragmatic, rooted in her practice of Reiki and responsive to the world around her.

HAWAYO TAKATA'S STORY OF REIKI

Some Reiki students were confused when, in the 1990s, contact with Japanese Reiki practitioners revealed that the story Takata told of how Reiki developed was not factual. Modern Americans and Europeans, disconnected from the functions stories play in indigenous cultures, didn't understand that Takata was a master storyteller who taught through demonstration and stories, both anecdotes of healings and her story of Reiki, which she spontaneously customized to the group in front of her. With a Hawaiian immigrant background and a life lived within the imported traditions of her parents' homeland, this type of communication, which Hawaiians call *talking story*,[10] was natural to her. Takata used her stories to impart understanding and, it seems, something more.

"Most of what Takata did was tell stories," Susan Mitchell told me. Mitchell learned First and Second Degree Reiki from Takata in 1978–79. She said, "As I sat there, I could feel the energy in the room build. I didn't have words for that. We didn't talk like that back then. As the class time progressed, I felt we were carried into another realm. I had a sense Takata had the ability to take us to a place where our own capacities would be awakened."

Takata's instruction was very concrete and specific, and she trusted her stories to carry the subtleties. Takata seemed convinced that the spirituality of Reiki would unfold naturally as students practiced over time, even without her specifying it.

Reiki master Susan Mitchell spent considerable time with Takata, who sometimes stayed at the Mitchells' home when she was teaching in California. (Takata insisted they start each day by giving each other hands-on treatment.) Mitchell says, "What Takata talked about depended upon whom she was with. In some groups, she spoke of more than physical healing." For Mitchell, however, the understanding that Reiki was not just about physical healing developed through her practice.

Although Takata did not stress this overtly, there is ample evidence that she valued Reiki as a spiritual healing practice. In a class Takata gave in California in the late 1970s, she said, "So we always say the mental and the spiritual is number one. Number two is the physical. And then you put that together and say we are a complete whole. And when you can say that, that means you have applied Reiki and Reiki has worked for you."[11] Takata sometimes referred to Reiki as "Godpower" (which she specified was universal and had no religious connotations), another indication that she saw Reiki as a spiritual healing practice.

Takata's mission was to transplant Reiki from its motherland and a culture that honored and protected it to a country that had never seen anything like it, where Reiki would be considered foreign and not necessarily viewed with respect. This was a particular challenge, given that the transition started in the late 1930s, a time of American isolationism and tense relations with Japan. Takata dedicated herself to ensuring that Reiki practice survived the tumultuous times.

As a direct result of that dedication, today Reiki is available throughout the world and is emerging as a viable healing practice in conventional medicine, a goal that Usui and Hayashi apparently supported.

By the time Takata died in December 1980, she had been practicing Reiki longer than Usui and Hayashi combined. For forty years, until she started training teaching masters in 1976, she had been the only Reiki master teaching in the West. In the four years before her death, she trained twenty-two Reiki masters. Her students faced life without their Reiki master with considerably less training time than Takata had had with Hayashi.

Takata spoke to several of her students about the possibility of carrying on her work, but she did not publicly announce any one of them as her successor. Although Takata's master students had scant contact among themselves during Takata's life, all but one of her master students now reached out for one another. Within a few years after Takata's death, most of the Reiki masters she had trained founded the Reiki Alliance and supported her granddaughter, Phyllis Lei Furumoto, in continuing Takata's work.

REIKI AFTER TAKATA

Within fifteen years of Takata's death, Reiki had spread from her twenty-two Canadian and American Reiki masters throughout the rest of the world. (Reiki continued to be taught in Japan by students of Usui and Hayashi. Japanese masters did not offer Reiki outside Japan and were not initially welcoming to the Western-trained masters who contacted them.) Takata practiced Reiki for forty years before training the bulk of her masters. But some of the masters Takata trained were training new masters within ten years of becoming masters themselves.

Takata's student Iris Ishikuro and Ishikuro's student Arthur Robertson began changing the practice and training masters less rigorously.[12] Rather than keeping Reiki as a separate practice, they also encouraged students to combine Reiki with New Age and other healing practices. The Reiki community quickly splintered into factions. Of course the masters who trained students rapidly created generations of students faster.

This was probably inevitable. The good news was that, bolstered by impressive anecdotal evidence and riding the crest of the New Age, Reiki proliferated rapidly.

But rapid proliferation also brought less stringent standards. How could rapid proliferation and respect for practice possibly coexist?

People who are totally new to Reiki can now take some form of master training in a weekend and teach others the next week. Many question this type of training. How can one teach others a practice that one has only just learned and not had time to actually practice? In what understanding and experience is this teaching rooted? Is "instant mastery" a basic contradiction in terms?

New Age advocates saw respect for practice and Takata as rigid, antiquated, even authoritarian. Students trained by Takata were flummoxed that anyone felt entitled to spread Takata's practice without regard for the standards and values she imparted. They didn't understand how students could ignore the necessity to practice, imagining that the initiation was everything, or feel authorized to change the practice on a whim. Such disregard of tradition seemed to them to dishonor both the woman who had championed the practice in America and Reiki itself.

For a while, Takata's students dug in their heels and engaged in a bit of navel gazing as they struggled to deepen their understanding and maintain Takata's tradition in the face of what felt like an onslaught of promiscuity in the practice. Reiki masters who had worked hard for their training and for whom becoming a master was a life-changing event watched Reiki mastery become devalued by those for whom it was another listing on a drop-down business card. Teaching standards and the roots of the practice were in danger of being lost. Before long, the traditionalists were outnumbered.

And yet Reiki as primordial consciousness is simply both subtler and more powerful than any system or form we may impose on it. This is not to say the system doesn't matter. It does. Systems are how wisdom traditions are passed along from generation to generation. A certain amount of change is inevitable and sometimes desirable, as when adapting details of a tradition to changing environments. Otherwise Reiki would never have left Japan. Such innovation is not made indiscriminately, but rather by master practitioners who have become rooted in the practice over years.

Reiki can certainly survive the fluidity that comes with years of disciplined practice, but if the initiations are passed to students and master candidates without respect and discipline, there would seem to be a point at which we don't know what, if anything, is happening.

As we know, people who hold themselves to high standards will always be vulnerable to accusations of elitism, and not without reason, while people who approach a subject in a less rigorous way tend to feel defensive around traditionalists. That is why it is important to create dialogue among Reiki masters of various lineages and practice styles that are focused on our commonality, so we can foster greater respect within this highly diverse community.

REIKI COMES HOME

There are many stamps on Reiki's originally Japanese passport. At its peak, the Reiki Alliance, the most conservative organization of Reiki masters, had one thousand members in over forty countries. It was inevitable in this age of globalization that Reiki would come full circle to reconnect with practitioners in Japan. As Western Reiki masters visited Japan, they eventually encountered the lineages of both Usui and Hayashi. Initially, the Japanese practitioners had no interest in how Reiki was practiced outside Japan, but over time, some interaction has taken place.

Because they had come to believe otherwise, many students were surprised as news of the existing Japanese students of Usui and Hayashi reached the West. The discrepancies between Takata's teaching stories and what continued in Japan didn't bother me at all. I can't second-guess the choices Takata made in bringing Reiki from Japan to a very foreign culture right before the United States went to war with Japan. Thanks to her devotion and commitment to Reiki, I am one of millions of people practicing Reiki today. I also felt complete in my practice and so was not looking for anything new to change or add to my own ever-expanding experience of Reiki.

Nonetheless, as information about Japanese students of Usui and Hayashi became available, I read it with interest, the way one might welcome news of a distant family member. I thought it unfortunate that the information was frequently bracketed by claims of authenticity and criticism toward Takata and even Hayashi. My understanding is that authenticity exists within our relationship to our practice—if we practice regularly with heartfelt commitment, our practice is authentic. All the same, I was delighted that what I learned about how Reiki is practiced in Japan was very validating to my practice, without changing it in any way.

For example, there was a time when, after many years of practice, my experience of Reiki was expanding beyond my training. At times, I felt Reiki's soft pulsations carried by my gaze. During treatment, I sometimes felt unusually condensed lasers of Reiki extending from my fingers. The expansion was rather sudden and so intense I wondered if this could still be Reiki. I continued to practice, observe, and contemplate. Since there was an unmistakable Reiki familiarity to what I experienced, I came to the conclusion that this was simply an organic expansion of Reiki.

Later, when I read about how Reiki was taught in the Japanese lineages of Usui and Hayashi, it was apparent that Japanese Reiki training included techniques similar to what had spontaneously developed out of my practice. This gave me great confidence in the power of the initiations when developed by consistent self-treatment. I should add that I have had similar experiences as I've learned more about Takata's practice. For example, I noticed early on that women with breast cancer drew Reiki strongly at the ovaries. Takata taught her students when treating women with lumps in the breast to treat the ovaries first and then the breast itself.[13]

Takata was a woman of pragmatic vision. She knew Reiki could not be transplanted wholesale from one culture to another, and that, with a watchful combination of steadiness and flexibility, Reiki would develop in a meaningful way in a new culture. Thanks to her foresight and courage, Reiki is thriving globally, albeit with a dizzying array of practice styles.

WHAT REIKI IS NOT

Beware of Reiki myths presented as fact. Reiki is often inaccurately referred to as a 2,500-year-old Buddhist tradition. In spite of documentation that Reiki practice was created by Mikao Usui, it is commonly misstated that he rediscovered the practice.

Others claim Reiki has come from the Medicine Buddha. This is ironic in that Tibetan Buddhists painstakingly trace their lineage of teachers back to the source of the practice. Believers may feel that all healing comes from the Medicine Buddha, and they may even have profound inner experiences of that, but we cannot make claims from inner experiences without tracing the lineage.

These myths may have stemmed from misunderstanding a comment Takata occasionally made, that Reiki (as *consciousness,* not as *practice*) was mentioned in 2,500-year-old Buddhist sutras. As discussed earlier, the term *Reiki* refers to both primordial consciousness and to this particular practice used to access primordial consciousness. Ancient Buddhist scripture refers to primordial consciousness only, not specifically to Reiki practice, which did not exist at the time. Reiki as a spiritual healing practice is neither ancient, nor Buddhist, nor Tibetan. Reiki practitioners are wise not to be roped in by unsubstantiated claims.

REIKI TODAY

As a Reiki master, I have been fortunate to have had the opportunity to create a number of hospital-based treatment and/or training programs in New York City hospitals, and to research many other such Reiki programs in the United States. The language and format of treatment often vary from what I use in my nonmedical practice (even in programs I have created), but the experience of Reiki is unvarying. As I help carry Reiki into conventional medicine, I often think of Takata and am inspired by her as a role model. Reiki has to stay simple if it is to integrate with conventional medicine, which is complicated enough. I have full confidence that just as Reiki managed the trip from Japan to America, Reiki can also weather transplantation into medical soil. It is proving to be fertile soil indeed.

Overall, then, there are currently three main branches of the Reiki lineage. The first is Usui, as brought forward by the Gakkai. The second is Usui/Hayashi. The third branch, Usui/Hayashi/Takata, has proliferated into styles that do not necessarily trace their lineage or resemble their common origin.*

Reiki's proliferation not only around the world but also into the conservative circles of conventional medicine bodes well for the future. My prayer is that rivalries among practitioners regarding authenticity will give way to respect for diversity. May there be Reiki plurality, with many dishes on the menu. May students freely choose the style of Reiki that appeals to them and meets their needs, which they will practice authentically. Mindful of our distinct practices, let us build on our commonalities and evidence our deep relationship with Reiki through the kindness and respect we extend to others.

---

*There are two Reiki masters teaching internationally who trace directly to the Japanese trunk of the Reiki family tree. Hyakuten Inamoto is a Buddhist monk who was trained by Chiyoko Yamaguchi, who studied First and Second Degree with Hayashi and was later trained as a Reiki master by one of Hayashi's master students. Inamoto is the founder of Komyo Reiki and president of the Komyo Reiki Association. Hiroshi Doi was originally trained in an offshoot of the Usui/Hayashi/Takata lineage, and later trained in the first two levels of practice by Kimiko Koyama (1906–1999), the sixth president of the Usui Reiki Ryoho Gakkai. He is a member of the Usui Reiki Ryoho Gakkai and a Reiki master, but he does not teach in the lineage of the Gakkai. Rather, Doi is the founder of Gendai Reiki Ho, and president of the Gendai Reiki Healing Association. He is the author of *Modern Reiki Method for Healing* (Fraser Journal Publishing, 2000).

Four

REIKI TREATMENT
OR TRAINING?

The most important thing is to find out what is the most important thing.

ZEN MASTER SHUNRYU SUZUKI

I have always loved being by the ocean. Whether I have hours to walk along the water's edge or just a few minutes to watch the rolling water, being by the ocean always changes my state for the better, imparting a feeling somewhat like a Reiki treatment. It's like a Reiki treatment in another way also: Once I'm in the right place, there's no more work for me to do but just be comfortable and let Reiki waft over me like the ocean air.

Like the ocean, the experience of Reiki is constant yet varied. Sometimes I feel amazing heat rise within me that can even make me break into a sweat. Other times, refreshing cool waves of pulsations flow throughout my body. And many Reiki experiences are less explicit than either of those extremes. I may feel suffused with well-being and relaxation, or sense gentle prickly vibrations either in my palms or under them, or in some other area of my body. I may be irresistibly drawn into a velvety deep inner state. What I notice depends on the situation and how much I'm inwardly paying attention.

If you're considering experiencing Reiki for yourself, you'll want to know more about the different possibilities open to you. You could make an appointment with a Reiki professional for a treatment. Or maybe you have a friend who has studied Reiki and would like to practice on you. Perhaps you are planning a hospital stay or are scheduled for a surgical procedure and have heard of Reiki being offered in your hospital, and are curious. All these are valid options, so let's look at each of them in detail. You may also be interested in taking a class and learning to practice Reiki on yourself (and your friend).

REIKI TREATMENT—WHAT TO EXPECT

Professional Treatment

A Reiki professional is just that—someone who supports herself financially by practicing Reiki on others. A professional will have a treatment space with a comfortable table where you lie on your back fully clothed, while she places her hands lightly on your head and the front of your torso. Eventually you'll be asked to turn on your stomach while your practitioner places hands on your back. (Some practitioners skip the back, which I think is a real loss. Be sure to tell your practitioner you would like Reiki hands on your back.) Different practitioners use somewhat different hand placements. Some practitioners place hands on the limbs as well as the head and torso. It's not so important exactly where Reiki hands are placed as long as none of the placements is invasive and you feel comfortable with what's happening. When receiving any kind of hands-on treatment, speak up immediately if touch is ever sexually inappropriate or even vaguely makes you uncomfortable. You needn't explain why; just ask the practitioner to move to the next placement. If a placement is uncomfortable for a client, a trustworthy professional will simply go on to the next placement without argument, trusting Reiki to do what needs to be done and what can be done to restore balance in the gentlest way possible.

A professional protects the treatment space from unnecessary interruptions and is prepared to respond to any special needs you have. For example, there is a point in pregnancy at which it is no longer advisable for the mother to lie flat on her back. A professional will accommodate a woman's needs at each stage of pregnancy by adapting positions, offering support with pillows or wedges, or using a comfortable chair. Be sure to mention any special needs when you make your appointment. Your session is your special time. By articulating your needs, you enable the practitioner to better serve you.

There may or may not be soft music playing during your Reiki session. Speak up if the selection or the volume doesn't suit you, or if you prefer silence. You may also want to bring your own music or recording of nature sounds. Clients often like to be covered during treatment regardless of the room temperature. Even if you don't feel the need when you start, ask if there is a blanket nearby in case you feel cool once you've settled down. Of course you don't want to disrupt the session unnecessarily, but don't be shy about requesting what you need to be comfortable. It is senseless and unnecessary to get up from the table with a backache when you could have asked for a bolster under your knees. And make any physical adjustments you need to during the session, including a trip to the bathroom.

Most people become very relaxed during even their first Reiki treatment, and the practitioner will give you ample time to "wake up" before you move off the table. There is usually time available for conversation about your experience, including any questions you may have about Reiki. You may also discuss when/if to have another treatment.

The length of professional sessions varies; somewhere between forty-five and ninety minutes is common. Reiki treatment from hospital staff is usually shorter, and only hand placements that are safely accessible are used, depending on the patient's condition and how many tubes are hooked up.

Practitioners have their own ways of conducting sessions, and often an initial session will start differently from subsequent sessions. Since I am not a medical professional, I do not take a medical history. Instead, I bring my client to the table right away. Once he's comfortably lying on his back, I rest my hand lightly at his solar plexus. This gives my client a chance to become familiar with my touch. I maintain relaxed eye contact while relating the logistics of the session and giving him a chance to tell me anything he wants me to know. I emphasize that his comfort is paramount to me and ask him to voice any needs that may arise during treatment, such as feeling chilly. I let my client know that when I finish, I'll leave the room briefly to get him a glass of filtered water, and ask him to remain lying down until I return to the room.

When my client is ready to sit up and talk, I elicit his description of the session. Putting words to the experience helps him remember it and provides a transition between the depth of the session and the rest of his day. The discussion naturally brings up any questions he might have pertaining to Reiki and issues of self-care. I am careful not to interpret my client's experience, even if he wants me to, as meaning is always up to the individual. This educational part of our session segues easily to any suggestions or information that might be useful to my client, or even referrals to other medical or healing practitioners.

Reiki is cumulative, and although you may experience great relief from the very first treatment, it is wise to have at least three or four sessions before evaluating what Reiki can do for you.

Although Reiki sessions are generally relaxing, don't assume that each session will be the same. Each session meets you where you are at that moment and moves you from that place closer to your unique place of balance. Sometimes this may take you into such a deep state that you wonder if you fell asleep. Other times you may hover between waking and sleeping, sensing many subtle shifts taking place throughout your being. Some sessions may fly by while others seem extended.

HOW MUCH TREATMENT?

If you're considering receiving Reiki treatment, you understandably want to know how quickly to expect results. Reiki practitioners cannot promise results any more than physicians can, but we can offer clients some guidelines. Remember always that Reiki encourages a person toward balance. Since each person is unique, each person will have a unique path to balance. Although each situation must be evaluated individually, acute conditions tend to balance faster than chronic conditions, and children tend to respond faster than adults (so much so that children's treatments can usually be modified).

I have never had a client go through an entire session without knowing that something had changed for the better. Reiki creates an immediate shift in one's state, but it also sets in motion subtle shifts that continue to develop over time. We cannot predict the path of healing, but we can watch. Although the experience of Reiki in each session is unique, drawn by the recipient according to what is needed in the moment, sessions tend to get noticeably stronger and deeper as treatment is continued.

Takata often treated people on four successive days. She felt this was a powerful way to jump-start the healing process. Reiki master Susan Mitchell finds treatment four days in a row to be much more profound than weekly treatment. I can't argue with this. However, the pace of urban and suburban life has accelerated since Takata died in 1980, and sometimes it just isn't possible even for people who are highly motivated to receive treatment four days in a row. And many people seek Reiki treatment without having the kind of health condition that warrants such focused attention. These savvy people are healthy and want to stay that way, and four consecutive treatments may seem unnecessary for maintenance. When clients ask me how many sessions they will need and how often, I tell them I really don't know until after I've given them a treatment. Generally speaking, however, someone who has a particular health condition is wise to start with at least a few sessions close together and then gradually space the sessions farther apart. Clients who learn Reiki and practice regularly on themselves usually need less frequent treatment from their practitioners.

After the initial treatment, before I make any recommendations, I ask my client what he would like to do. Often we're thinking along the same lines. If not, I'll try to gently steer him toward my assessment, but without making demands, mindful of Takata's words "Do what you can. Some Reiki is better than none at all."[1]

As clients experience benefits from Reiki, feeling better and functioning more easily, they often become more motivated to receive treatment and even to learn Reiki themselves. Once trained, clients can self-treat as much as they like. Additionally, they will draw Reiki even more strongly when they return for professional treatment.

My mother often said, "God helps those who help themselves." It certainly has been my experience with Reiki. The client who is willing to learn Reiki and self-treat definitely has the best results, but I never pressure clients to take the training. People come to it in their own time, and some just don't.

People with serious illnesses are sometimes advised to do what I call Reiki marathons, which come in two varieties. Clients either come for treatment every day for an extended time (twenty-one days is common), or a group of practitioners and/or students gathers to give the patient all-day treatment. In the latter situation, the patient lies on the table for hours at a time (with comfort breaks) while practitioners show up to join the treatment team as they are available. Either of these options can give wonderful results and may be desirable, especially if it can be arranged with some ease, but in my experience, they may not be necessary if the patient is self-treating daily and receiving treatment regularly and frequently from another practitioner. There is something to be said for giving the body time to fully digest the treatment, which really doesn't end when Reiki hands are lifted.

Physicians can't predict how a particular patient will respond to measured doses of a specific medication that has been tested for efficacy. So how can we predict how much Reiki treatment an individual will need? Reiki can't be quantified. We don't know how much Reiki anyone gets in a session; we only know that people precipitate what Reiki they need in the present time, in the way they can best integrate it, according to the ability of the practitioner. I have seen many clients heal by receiving treatment within their financial and scheduling parameters. In deciding how much treatment you need, follow your intuition and work in the way that serves you on every level. How much treatment you need depends on a lot of variables, and can change abruptly. There may be a week in which you feel you need an extra treatment. That doesn't mean you need to continue at that pace. Although everyone likes a schedule, and there are many benefits to receiving Reiki regularly, you can be flexible and creative.

Reiki is not just for those in crisis. I encourage clients to come for treatment on a regular basis, even if it's twice a year at the turn of the seasons. Treatment in spring and fall brings balance as the body adjusts to climatic changes. Not only is the treatment pleasurable, but it also does much to strengthen well-being and prevent illness.

HOW WILL I KNOW IF REIKI
IS HELPING ME?

Some people are quite confident deciding whether something works for them or not. Even without having immediate and dramatic changes, they sense a positive shift in their overall experience of themselves and of life that they know will lead to desirable results. If this is not true for you, consider keeping a journal to help you evaluate what is emerging from your Reiki treatment. You'll want to record both the immediate experience and what you notice overall. This journal is just for you, so make it easy to do. You needn't use full sentences, and it doesn't even have to be verbal. You could draw faces to indicate how you feel, like the smiley, neutral, and frowny faces used to indicate pain in hospitals. However you choose, be sure to make notes of how you feel before and after each session. Take a few minutes before bed to reflect on your day, reviewing your mood and mental clarity, your steadiness, your productiveness, your social interactions, and anything else that was part of why you went for treatment. For example, if insomnia drove you to Reiki, each morning, note how you slept. Did you fall asleep easily? Did you stay asleep? What was the quality of your sleep? Did you awaken refreshed? If you woke during the night, did you go back to sleep easily? You can make a simple numbered scale and rate yourself each day so you can look back over a month and see if there has been improvement. See the VAS scale illustrated on page 216.

Ultimately, we all have to decide for ourselves what heals us and what is our ability to make it part of our lives. Something that helps us simply feel better is valuable. Relaxation is not a luxury; it is a biochemical event and a medical necessity. Life is chockfull of stressors, and countless stimuli are continually amping up our systems. Even machines have to stop for care and maintenance, and people often take better care of their cars than they do of themselves, largely because they don't know how to care for themselves. Reiki can fill that need.

Informal Treatment

Perhaps you have a friend or family member who has learned Reiki. Even a student who has just completed the First Degree training is able to share Reiki informally and is usually grateful for an opportunity to practice on someone else. Although the overall experience of a friendly treatment may lack the polish and accommodation of a professional treatment, receiving Reiki from someone you know can be a lovely experience if you are comfortable being touched by that person. Realize that your friend may feel unsure of herself or even a little shy, especially if she is new to the practice, and may not have the experience to structure the situation and take care of your needs the way a professional would. She may not yet even know how to take care of her own needs.

Nonetheless, if you are comfortable enough with each other and have a sense of adventure, once the treatment starts you will both relax and have a very pleasant experience. It is pleasurable and uplifting to offer Reiki, so don't worry that your friend is sacrificing her well-being for you. In fact, she is also receiving healing as she gives a treatment. Because Reiki emanates from the subtlest source within us, it refreshes the practitioner as well as the person being treated.

The main difference between treating yourself and treating someone else is that you need to stay awake while you're treating someone else—unless, of course, it's someone who shares your bed! This is a strong point of agreement across diverse styles of Reiki. With Reiki, the difference between practitioner and recipient is mostly a matter of which role they play during treatment, not who's getting a healing.

If neither you nor your practitioner friend has a professional table, you can improvise a treatment space on a studio couch (one without arms), on a bed that doesn't have a footboard, or, with sufficient padding, on a large dining table. It's also possible to have a modified chair session of Reiki. In this case your friend may not be placing hands on all the areas used in a full treatment, but even ten to fifteen minutes of having Reiki hands on your head, upper chest, and perhaps the upper back can be quite wonderful (see the Appendix). If the relationship is comfortable, informal sharing of Reiki can be very effective. This was how I was introduced to Reiki, and my first experience inspired me to call my friend's Reiki master and learn to practice First Degree Reiki the very next week!

Hospital Treatment

It is also possible that you may be offered Reiki by a staff member during a hospital visit, perhaps before or after surgery or chemotherapy. Hospital sessions are usually considerably shorter than private sessions, often lasting between fifteen to twenty minutes, or even less. Hospital personnel tend to use fewer hand placements for a number of reasons—time limitations, access to the patient's body is blocked by tubes and medical apparatus, or the patient can't be turned. You may be asked to fill out a feedback form to document your experience. If you are in a hospital or conventional health-care facility for any reason and you have a visitor who knows Reiki, he can offer you Reiki either as a full treatment (if he can get around the medical equipment) or simply by placing a hand anywhere that's accessible and comfortable for both of you.

You can also arrange for your own Reiki practitioner—a friend or a professional—to give you Reiki treatment during your hospital stay. Besides giving treatment to clients of all ages in their hospital rooms, I have also offered Reiki during chemotherapy, in surgical holding areas before surgery, in operating rooms during surgery, in intensive-care units after surgery or during various medical crises, and in labor and delivery. I have never run into resistance from medical staff. If a physician comes in while I'm giving a treatment, I offer to step aside, but usually the doctor insists I continue. Physicians and nurses often have to hurt the patient in order to help (even having a wound carefully dressed can be painful), and they appreciate gentle care that brings their patient peace. Sometimes the nurse or doctor asks to observe, in which case I offer to place my hand on his head or shoulder so he can feel Reiki.

Reiki Self-Treatment

Sometimes it isn't possible or even desirable to receive treatment from someone else, especially if there are financial concerns or no Reiki friend is available. Don't worry— I have trained many students in First Degree who had not experienced Reiki treatment, and it has never created an obstacle to learning.

Receiving Reiki either from oneself or from another person is effective, although the overall experience and the specific advantages are a little different. On the one hand, being taken care of by someone else is a wonderful and multileveled experience. But it takes some arranging and scheduling, and if it is a professional appointment, there's a fee. On the other hand, once you learn to practice Reiki, help is literally never farther away than the end of your arm. There's no scheduling, no additional fee, and no wait. This is an advantage to anyone, but especially to parents, children, and anyone with chronic pain or illness. For many people, it makes (dollars and) sense to avoid the treatment fee and to spend their money directly to learn to practice Reiki for self-treatment, an investment that yields dividends for life.

There are myriad other reasons why people may prefer self-treatment. Anyone who is shy about touch either because of trauma or abuse or simply personal preference may want to go straight to class to learn Reiki practice themselves. If you are considering learning Reiki without any prior experience, be assured that as long as you take the time to find a competent teacher, there is no disadvantage in treating yourself. There are even data to back up that claim. Students in my hospital-based HIV classes filled out anonymous questionnaires rating pain and anxiety before and after receiving a twenty-minute Reiki treatment from either themselves or another student. All these students were people who were HIV+ and receiving their medical care at an inner-city clinic. (These data were collected during the third and fourth sessions of a four-day class, so these students were really brand-new practitioners.) Using rating scales that have proven accuracy and are used in research, we found that both the students who received treatment from another student *and* those who treated themselves experienced a significant reduction in both anxiety and pain.

LEVELS OF REIKI TRAINING AND PRACTICE

I will go over the different levels of Reiki training in greater detail in the chapters to come, but a brief overview here will provide the basics. Takata offered three levels of training, each preparing the student for a particular aspect of practice.

First Degree Reiki is healing through proximity, either hands-on, light touch, or, when medically indicated, hands just above an open wound or burn. Since First Degree students learn hands-on self-treatment, the foundation of Reiki practice at all levels, this is all the training that most people need.

Second Degree is distant, nontouch healing.

The third level of Reiki training is to become a Reiki master. Traditionally, this has meant a commitment to initiate and train students to practice Reiki, which only Reiki masters can do.

Although training is available at the above levels, it's important to understand that we develop our relationship with Reiki through practice, not by taking more classes. I have met First Degree students who practiced daily self-treatment and were more profoundly engaged with Reiki than many Reiki masters.

INITIATION—A BEGINNING WITHOUT END

Initiations, the core of Reiki training, create alignment in the student's biofield, the subtle vibrational field that surrounds, penetrates, and supports the physical body, which enables the student to practice Reiki. Since only a qualified Reiki master can give these initiations, which are sometimes referred to as empowerments or attunements, all levels of Reiki practice are taught only by Reiki masters.

You will receive four initiations for First Degree training and one for Second Degree. All initiations will take place during the Reiki class. When it is time for the initiation, your Reiki master will either come to each student individually or take each student into another room. You will sit comfortably, eyes closed, palms together in front of your forehead while the Reiki master spends a short time at the crown of your head and then with your hands.

The initiations as Takata taught them were primarily an inner experience; the outward ritual was rather simple. In the years since Takata's death, some Reiki masters have further embellished the process. Although additions are not necessary, they need not pose a problem as long as the core process has not been corrupted.

During initiation, many students have a subtle (or not-so-subtle) sense of opening, as if an inner door leads into a great expanse, or a palpable sense of freedom. Other students experience nothing but notice a difference in their hands afterward. I often compare the initiation process to a subtle chiropractic adjustment. I'm not sure exactly what happened during the adjustment, but I can tell that there is greater ease as a result and—most important—I feel better.

Because of the initiation process, in which the Reiki master literally jump-starts your practice, anyone who chooses to be trained is able to practice Reiki, and I mean anyone. The empowerments make the subtle connections that allow healing Reiki pulsations to activate in the practitioner's hands, directly from unlimited primordial consciousness. The initiations enable the Reiki student to carry Reiki potential in her hands that can activate spontaneously according to the need of anyone she touches, herself or another.

When you contact the unified field and when I contact the unified field, it's the same unified field we're connected to. All that varies is the connection itself, which will be unique to the individual. Each of us is unique, and our connection to Reiki and our relationship with Reiki will also be unique. Some people are more temperamentally inclined toward Reiki. Some Reiki masters are more effective than others, making their initiations more powerful. And some people simply practice more than others. These three variables affect our connection to Reiki: the student's innate talent, the effectiveness of the empowerments, and continuing practice.

I have been initiated into two lineages of Reiki, both by Reiki masters whose Reiki masters had been trained by Takata. It was apparent to me that all the initiations I received were effective. Not only did I experience something in the initiation process, but also the change in my hands was unmistakable.

However, not everyone feels as immediate and powerful a connection to Reiki as I did. If you are disappointed in your experience of Reiki training and, despite having practiced sincerely, don't feel that anything is happening in your hands, there is no harm in approaching another master for training and being initiated again.

The reason people can benefit from Reiki self-treatment whether they are a little off center (many of us!) or even seriously ill is because after a person has been initiated, Reiki pulsates spontaneously from its universal source, primordial consciousness, which is also called Reiki. When someone is ill or even just "off his game," there is a disturbance in his biofield. Sometimes people, especially those addressing chronic illness, are concerned that "their Reiki" won't be good enough. There is no need for concern. Because Reiki is primordial consciousness, everyone's Reiki is essentially the same. It's pure, pristine, pulsating consciousness, and we all can access it. Many people have spontaneous experiences of a benevolent reality that seems to both contain the ordinary and exist beyond it. This is primordial consciousness, that sea of awareness that permeates the inner and outer realities. Very advanced meditators and spiritual adepts of all traditions can connect with primordial consciousness at will. For the rest of us—those who haven't devoted our lives to spiritual pursuits—the Reiki initiations are a major leg up. They give us the ability to access primordial consciousness reliably, effectively, and spontaneously, without having to focus or change our state or call it forth or even remember it. This is an obvious boon in an emergency or in the face of serious illness, but it's also a great boon in everyday life.

The initiations at each level of practice are to open the student to that scope of practice. They do not, however, replace the deepening that comes only through consistent practice over time. We've all seen what can happen when people get promoted too quickly or when a skyrocketing early career short-circuits maturity. I haven't heard a convincing argument why Reiki practice is any different. And why would someone want to move quickly through all levels of initiation? It seems to imply a lack of recognition of what is accomplished by initiation. The initiations themselves are subtle and take mere moments to enact; their effects take a lifetime to develop. What is gained by fast-tracking spirituality? Is it even possible to do so? With all due respect to "the fast-food nation," is it possible that the person who receives all levels of initiation at one sitting digests the effects as well as if the initiations were spaced over (considerable) time? A person who is using Reiki primarily for self-care may not consider this an issue worth contemplating. He's happy to know he needs only First Degree training. But this discussion is very relevant to someone using Reiki with others. When we assume the responsibility to treat or teach others, inadequate training and experience can be a liability to the well-being of both practitioner and receiver. Committed daily practice yields the best results for any student of Reiki, and daily self-treatment becomes even more important when one is treating or teaching others, anchoring the practitioner in the practice of self-care that is the foundation of Reiki.

PRACTICE

We are all equal in essence, but we are also unique, and there is no equality in the details of our uniqueness. So of course some people will be comfortable with Reiki faster than others. But the speed with which one feels proficient with Reiki doesn't matter. What matters is that the student practice Reiki consistently. In my experience, the differences in the speed with which students learn Reiki do not predict their ultimate relationship with the practice. Sometimes people find Reiki so simple that they don't bother to practice and totally miss how profound it is. Other students may feel Reiki isn't an easy fit initially, but they commit themselves to daily practice. As their discomfort dissolves over time, their love of the practice grows, and Reiki becomes an important support in their lives.

One of my students at Gay Men's Health Crisis was a former college professor from Chile who had lost his job and his home as a result of his AIDS diagnosis. Eduardo was in such poor health and feeling so hopeless that he came to the Reiki class out of sheer desperation and with no clear sense of what he actually would be doing in the class. Reiki was unlike anything this academic had ever experienced, and his intellect was in no hurry to admit something was happening during a Reiki session.

But Eduardo had achieved his academic success through hard work, and he brought the same work ethic to Reiki. One of the most intelligent and accomplished students I've taught, Eduardo was also the slowest in other ways! But he kept practicing, and eventually his analytical mind accepted what was happening.

Although Eduardo has had many health challenges over the years, he has persisted in his Reiki practice and remained open to supporting his well-being in every way available to him, including acupuncture and conventional medicine. Four years after his First Degree class, Eduardo became a Second Degree student. Years later, his health is good, he is once again employed as an academic, and he has become an American citizen. He continues to practice Reiki every day. Who would ever have guessed that Reiki would become so important to someone who felt completely out of his element in the First Degree class?

Just as I have witnessed Eduardo's growth over the years, I have also seen many "gifted" students come and go. They notice the sensations of Reiki quite easily but lack either the understanding or the discipline to develop their talent through regular practice. So if you are interested in learning Reiki, please put aside any concern that your Reiki won't be "good enough." Find a teacher who suits you (more on how to do this in the next chapter), start your practice, and never stop. Don't be defeated by perfectionism. With Reiki, the only mistake you can make is not to practice.

Five

FINDING AND CHOOSING YOUR REIKI CONNECTION

Better too skeptical than too trusting.

CHINESE PROVERB

You might be considering Reiki because a friend found that Reiki helped relieve his depression. Or maybe your mother's neighbor is sleeping better since her daughter began giving her treatment. Maybe you've always been interested in spirituality or intrigued by subtle energies, but everything attached to either of them seemed too far-out. Perhaps you're sensitive to drugs and want to find a gentler way to relieve assorted aches and pains, or you're wary of medications and going to the doctor for every little thing and want something you can do for yourself. Maybe you're not getting the results you expected from psychotherapy and you're sick of talking but realistic enough to know you could be feeling better about yourself.

People come to Reiki for countless and varied reasons, and some people don't have a reason other than just feeling drawn to it. Chapter 4 has helped you decide whether you want to receive a treatment from someone else or if you want to learn to practice

Reiki yourself. Now let's help you find a practitioner, if you want a treatment, or a Reiki master, if you want a class.

FINDING A REIKI PRACTITIONER OR A REIKI MASTER

If you want to receive treatment rather than learn to practice yourself, you need to find a Reiki practitioner trained in First or Second Degree practice. Because there are no uniform standards for Reiki training, it's impossible to judge a practitioner's skill by her level of certification. First Degree students can actually have more training than some Reiki masters (just to refresh your memory, First Degree practice is hands-on, Second Degree includes distant healing as well as hands-on, but only Reiki masters can both give treatment and initiate students into the practice). Although everyone can learn to practice Reiki, some people will have more innate talent as healers. However, committed students will more than make up for lack of talent and training by devoting themselves to the consistent practice of Reiki self-treatment. So if you are looking for someone to give you Reiki treatment, don't sweat the level, just look for credible practitioners at any level—First Degree, Second Degree, or Reiki master.

If you've decided you want to learn to practice Reiki, First or Second Degree practitioners can't help you. You can only learn Reiki practice from a qualified Reiki master, and traditionally, Reiki training has taken place in person. However, a First or Second Degree Reiki practitioner can tell you who trained him, and that may be a good place to start looking for a Reiki class.

But you might decide to learn Reiki without ever having experienced a treatment. You may have personal or financial reasons to skip treatment and go right to class. After all, once you've learned Reiki, you can give yourself treatment as often as you like, for as long as you want. People with serious illness often practice Reiki self-treatment many times a day. Its simplicity and flexibility make that possible even for people with low energy and busy schedules, such as those who continue working while undergoing chemotherapy. And self-treatment brings results quickly.

THE REIKI ALLIANCE

No matter whether you are looking for treatment or training, for a Reiki practitioner or a Reiki master, the Reiki Alliance can be a good resource. The Alliance is a professional organization of Reiki masters committed to Takata's legacy.* Their website (www.reikialliance.com) lists the worldwide membership with contact information.[1] Whether or not there is an Alliance master in your immediate vicinity, the nearest one can likely recommend a student close by who offers treatment, or even a Reiki circle in your area.

Reiki circles or clinics are gatherings in which Reiki practitioners share modified or full treatments with one another and with community members, usually as community service or on a donation basis. Attending a Reiki circle in your area gives you an opportunity to experience Reiki and to connect with local practitioners.

If you are looking for Reiki classes, a master you locate through the Reiki Alliance will have a similar perspective to what this book expresses. Although Alliance masters are committed to Takata's legacy, they are each masters in their own right, and there will be individual variation in what it means to practice à la Takata. Each master has his or her own experience and understanding and draws the line in different places. The individuality of their practice styles has most likely evolved out of prolonged practice. The masters in Reiki Alliance received their training slowly and usually had the benefit of extended mentoring. They also participate in the global community of Alliance masters as they are able, benefiting from that support and stimulation.

Another seek-and-find strategy is to ask a respected health-care professional who

---

* After becoming a Reiki master, I waited nearly three years to join the Reiki Alliance. Although I support the goal of upholding Takata's values in our practice, I am also sensitive to unnecessary regulation. After many long talks with members and much contemplation, my understanding is that the Reiki Alliance seeks to keep a balance between maintaining Takata's practice and honoring individual mastery. I am not a spokesperson for the Reiki Alliance, and everything expressed in this book is my own understanding.

practices a complementary or alternative (CAM) modality such as acupuncture or shiatsu if she can recommend a Reiki practitioner. Getting into the local network of CAM providers will likely lead you to a Reiki practitioner who carries Reiki credibly enough to be respected by her professional community. Also, your local hospital may offer Reiki to inpatients or host a community Reiki circle, clinic, or training.

Churches or local continuing-education programs sometimes offer Reiki circles, so look in the service listings in your neighborhood paper. Scope out the local health-food store for notices or directories of local health practitioners. And don't forget to put the word out among your circle of friends. You might be surprised who else is interested in or already knows about Reiki.

Don't limit yourself to finding a Reiki master in your immediate area. If you are a natural enthusiast who can easily gather friends for an event, you might be able to attract a Reiki master to your area by organizing a class of your friends.

CHOOSING A REIKI PRACTITIONER OR REIKI MASTER

Your search may have brought you to more than one Reiki practitioner, or you may find a number of Reiki masters teaching in your area. How to choose one, especially if you've never experienced Reiki, might seem puzzling. Let's simplify the process.

First of all, eschew the thinking that there is one best practitioner or master. Thinking there is a "best doctor," "best acupuncturist," "best massage therapist," "best Reiki practitioner" is not helpful. It's actually misleading. Many professionals are well trained and experienced, and practice with integrity. The question, instead, should be: Who best suits my unique needs? The answer to this is often simply the practitioner or master to whom you feel most drawn from among those who meet your criteria. But in case it's not that simple, read on. The choice of a Reiki practitioner differs somewhat from that for a Reiki master and class, so we'll look at them separately.

CHOOSING A REIKI PRACTITIONER FOR TREATMENT

When possible, it's an advantage to choose a practitioner close at hand. Going out of your way for an occasional treatment or to take Reiki training is one thing, but you won't want to travel a long distance on a regular basis, especially if you're not feeling well.

It is reasonable to have a brief phone conversation with a practitioner before booking an appointment. This is your chance to ask about the practitioner's training and get a sense of her personality. There is no yardstick for measuring a Reiki practitioner, but you can learn a lot by asking the following questions:

1. When did you complete each level of training, and how many hours of instruction did it involve? Longer training is probably more thorough, especially if the student takes ample time to practice before training at the next level.

2. Were you physically present with the Reiki master giving the initiations? Although distant initiations may be justified in extenuating circumstances, there are many advantages to being initiated by a physically present Reiki master. Students who have received initiations through the Internet may have not gotten any training at all.

3. Do you practice daily self-treatment? Self-treatment is the foundation of Reiki at all levels and the discipline that matures our understanding.

4. What clinical experience have you had since your training—e.g., approximately how many treatments have you given and in what circumstances (private practice, hospital, etc.)? If you are receiving Reiki from a friend, it doesn't particularly matter if you are the first person he treats. If, however, you are seeking a professional, it's reasonable to look for someone with years of experience.

5. How do you describe Reiki? It's important that a professional be able to communicate the practice clearly and credibly without making claims or

disparaging conventional medicine. The answer to this question will tell you a lot about the practitioner's understanding of Reiki, how she carries the practice, and whether she would be able to collaborate with your physician, in case that becomes desirable.

6. What can I expect during your session? Do you include practices other than Reiki in your sessions? You deserve a quick run-through, particularly to know how long the session will be and to ensure that the treatment involves only Reiki (this is often important to people, particularly for medical reasons). Make sure that you will not be asked to disrobe. Reiki treatment is given through clothing.

7. What is your unique perspective as a Reiki practitioner? Again, this is an opportunity to learn about the practitioner. For example, my unique perspective is that I have over forty years of spiritual practice and that I collaborate frequently with medical professionals. Someone looking for a practitioner with experience collaborating with physicians might be interested in working with me.

8. What is your fee and how is it to be paid? Do you have a cancellation policy?

Asking about lineage or style may or may not yield information. The oft-heard term Usui Reiki doesn't carry any standard understanding or practice guidelines. Many practitioners say they practice Usui Reiki without knowing what it means, just because that's what they were told. And there are many fine Reiki practitioners who cannot trace their lineage back to Takata but who practice diligently and have a deep, mature relationship with Reiki. There are also practitioners who trace their lineage to Takata but don't mention (and often don't know) how much the practice they learned has been changed from the practice Takata taught. Even Reiki Alliance masters might take latitude in their practice, so if you have specific desires or expectations, ask specific questions. It is best not to assume anything.

It is worthwhile to ask the above questions even if the Reiki practitioner has other health-care credentials, perhaps as a nurse or a massage therapist. Whereas professionals who have other health-care training are more likely to be skilled when it comes to important details of clinical practice such as when medical care is needed, they may actually be less skilled and experienced in giving full Reiki treatment. A health-care provider who is trained to actively intervene may find it difficult to sit in silence and allow Reiki to accomplish the healing. So asking how much experience he has giving full Reiki treatment is a good idea.

Additionally, health-care professionals are often less at ease with individual variations in healing than lay practitioners are. Compare the different ways in which an obstetrician and a midwife support a woman in labor: The physician is confined to a narrower set of expectations defined in standard medical practice and intervenes readily. The midwife has a wider tolerance for each woman's individual process, relies more on watchful waiting, and intervenes only when needed.

REIKI, SPIRITUALITY, AND RELIGION

Whereas religion involves shared beliefs and dogma, spirituality is an individual, inner dialogue with the unseen that may include specific practices such as meditation or prayer. A Reiki practitioner's specific religious beliefs aren't important (within reason), but the ongoing inner engagement we call spiritual practice is transformational and dovetails powerfully with Reiki practice. A longstanding and regular spiritual practice softens the edges of the mind's tendency toward criticism and judgment. Spiritual practice develops compassion, respect, and gratitude for the power of Reiki, and healthy boundaries.

Meditation in particular is a natural companion to Reiki, rather like an inner practice of Reiki, in which the pulsations are traced back to the source. The practice of meditation helps develop the inner awareness and the ability to sit and be centered that are so valuable in a Reiki practitioner. Two excellent books on meditation from the SYDA Foundation that discuss vibration are Swami Durgananda (Sally Kempton)'s *The Heart of Meditation* (Siddha Yoga Publications, 2002) and Swami Shantananda's *The Splendor of Recognition* (Siddha Yoga Publications, 2003).

JUST REIKI, PLEASE

Some practitioners offer a dizzying array of techniques in their treatment sessions. Although this can be impressive, especially to someone who is exploring Reiki or holistic healing for the first time, I prefer to work with a practitioner who has immersed herself in the practice and who is comfortable with silence. I've never found this inner grounding in a practitioner who gets involved with problem solving using a lot of different techniques. Such practitioners have explained to me that they use Reiki for this and that and another technique for something else, a third technique for whatever, and so on. I'm not saying this is wrong; however, my experience has been that Reiki can address all those needs in a very simple, straightforward way, if allowed to. Rather than a mélange of techniques, which frequently includes the practitioner's voice, I enjoy the silence and depth of a Reiki treatment that is just that—a Reiki treatment.

Practitioners who move quickly through their training may lack the patience needed to be good clinicians, rushing to fix problems and controlling clients' healing paths rather than facilitating and relying on watchful waiting. Experienced massage therapists, however, may offer clients a range of techniques to match the range of bodies and preferences for touch that clients bring. They may use Reiki briefly before and/or after the active part of the massage to deeply relax clients and create harmony between client and therapist. This is an effective use of Reiki, but it is still a massage, not a Reiki session. If you are looking for a Reiki session, make sure that is what you are going to get. If the practitioner hems and haws, or tries to talk you into anything, look elsewhere.

TIME TO CHOOSE

As you evaluate the information you've gathered, reflect on your own values. This part of the process may not be different from how you would choose a physician, if you have the luxury of choice. Some people prize training and reputation, and gravitate toward the wall with the most diplomas, citations, and press clippings (remember that unlike medical certificates, Reiki certificates can be acquired on the Internet, so be sure to inquire). Others value clinical manner as highly as training. I lean in that direction, especially for low-tech Reiki. What I value most is a practitioner who gives himself Reiki every day.

There is also a great advantage in receiving treatment—and especially Reiki training—from someone who has a committed spiritual practice in addition to a daily practice of Reiki self-treatment. Practice is where the rubber meets the road, and having a daily spiritual practice distinguishes a Reiki practitioner from someone who simply talks spiritually or who only goes to an occasional meditation group or chanting concert. Having a spiritual practice means a person takes responsibility for his spiritual well-being and engages with his spirituality on a daily basis. The form of the practice doesn't matter; it might be meditation or prayer, t'ai chi, qigong, or yoga—the list of possibilities is long—but taking time every day to be alone with oneself creates an inner anchor that makes a healer both steadier and more powerful. If I wanted to learn to play golf, I would find someone who golfs every day. Why settle for less when learning or experiencing Reiki?

Once you have gathered the information you need, proceed on the basis of your gut. You may be lucky enough to find several competent practitioners. Go with the one you like the best, the one with whom you feel most at ease.

Reiki treatment is a pleasurable experience that can become a cherished haven in your life. Trust yourself enough to go with the practitioner to whom you feel most drawn, even if he does not have the most training and/or clinical experience. If Reiki is a rainbow, each practitioner is a lens through which a portion of the rainbow can be accessed, and there may be no practitioner through whom the entire spectrum shines. A wide-spectrum practitioner has a lot to offer, but that may be less important if what you need most is deep purple. Few people can analyze such needs. Trust your intuition.

You may or may not stay with the first Reiki practitioner you choose. As we heal, our needs change. Your intuition may lead you elsewhere, and that's fine. It's not an indictment of either you or the practitioner. Or you may like Reiki but not like the practitioner's style so much. I do not hesitate to refer a prospective client to a colleague if my sense is that we are not a good match, but it took years to develop that confidence. If you're not thrilled with your practitioner, try someone else before you give up on Reiki.

CHOOSING A REIKI MASTER AND CLASS

With the rapid proliferation of Reiki throughout the world since Takata's death in 1980, Reiki classes now come in a wide array of formats, fees, and styles to suit everyone from the strict traditionalist to the New Age avant-gardist. With such an array of class formats, fees, and styles of Reiki, how can a potential student make a good choice? What matters most is finding a teacher who meets your criteria for competency and whom you like, who teaches classes in a format that fits your circumstances. The questions to ask when choosing a Reiki practitioner (see page 74) are also useful when interviewing Reiki masters. Ask masters about their teaching experience as well as their clinical experience. Since Reiki is practical rather than theoretical, a Reiki master with considerable clinical experience in Reiki has a stronger foundation for teaching.

Some Reiki masters teach very much as Takata did, in four sessions on successive days. This can be arranged as either one session per day over four successive days or with sessions doubled up over a weekend. In the latter case, a class might start Friday evening, have two sessions on Saturday, and end with a session on Sunday. Or there may be two sessions each on Saturday and Sunday. Although the immersion of this format can make the class seem like a retreat, it doesn't provide support for taking your practice home, especially if the Reiki master leaves town after class.

Although I will always custom-design a class, arranging the ten to twelve hours of class time to suit a particular need, I usually teach in three four-hour sessions scheduled over a week. This arrangement gives students time between sessions to practice at home. Students then return to class with the questions that come up only when we practice outside class. By the time class is over, students are already in their second week of daily self-treatment. This format supports my primary goal as a Reiki master, which is to launch students into their lifelong Reiki practice. I also find it works well for the hyper-scheduled New Yorkers I teach, who rarely have four consecutive evenings available. Mothers, especially those who work outside the home, find it particularly difficult to be out four nights in a row.

One-day classes are a common option. They typically include less than ten hours of actual class time, which may work for small groups. Depending on the Reiki master, a one-day immersion can create a sense of a retreat, which is a plus for people who don't usually take even a day to devote to their well-being. The retreat aspect of the class alone is healing, and you go home with a skill for life. Single-day classes, however, do not offer support to students as they take Reiki into their lives, especially if taught by a traveling Reiki master. Although I experimented with one-day classes as I began teaching Reiki, I now use that format only if it is the sole arrangement available, such as when I teach at a medical conference. In that situation, I offer students ongoing e-mail support.

Even in a single-day class, I give each of the four initiations separately, with as much time between them as possible. Some Reiki masters teaching in a day or less "save time" by giving the initiations either all at once or two and two. The initiations and practice are the core of Reiki training. Their value is such that anything else that happens during the class needs to be worked into a time frame that supports them. Grouping the initiations to squeeze them into the schedule discounts their value and doesn't allow the student time to integrate each initiation. Just as a lifesaving injection takes seconds to administer, Reiki initiations take only moments to accomplish. Both begin processes that continue to play out in the individual's system, and it is naive not to honor that timing. There may be rare situations in which a megadose is the best option, but generally giving each initiation separately supports maximum effectiveness and smoothest integration.

Some Reiki masters offer First Degree classes in a single afternoon or evening. Others offer First and Second Degree, or even master training, all in one class. That doesn't leave much time for covering the material, never mind providing enough practice time so students leave with the knowledge that something has actually happened. As Reiki masters, we are not simply empowering the practice but also supporting students to actually start practicing. It's likely that short classes like these include only one initiation, not the four Takata used. For these reasons, should you wish to go on to Second Degree Reiki or even become a Reiki master, I recommend taking your time.

CYBER REIKI

I have stumbled onto websites that promise distant initiation, sometimes through the Internet, usually with no fee. I would suggest that the prospective student simply consider if this is the best way for him to learn Reiki. The price may be appealing, and this option certainly simplifies scheduling, but does it truly meet the student's needs? At best, Internet learning of this type offers no support. My experience is that most people learn this type of material best through interacting face-to-face with a Reiki master and with other people in class.

REIKI AND MONEY

In truth, Reiki is not for sale. The fees we pay Reiki professionals are to compensate for their time so that Reiki is given and received as part of a balanced interaction that respects client and practitioner alike. When we receive Reiki from a beginning student, the opportunity to give treatment is payment enough.

The fees Reiki practitioners charge are a reflection of their own understanding and experience with Reiki and healing itself, their sense of value, and practicalities such as the local cost of living.

Make a realistic appraisal of your finances and decide the range that you are comfortable spending. Cost of treatment may factor into your decision of where to receive treatment or whether to learn to self-treat. The range of fees for treatment varies enormously, especially among different locales. Even with the full realization that what you learn in a Reiki class is yours for life, you may have very real financial restraints. All students need to evaluate the situation for themselves.

Consider the experience of the Reiki master and the number of hours (this is one aspect where more probably *is* better) when comparing fees for classes. The size of the class may also figure in. Class format and logistics can add costs in terms of travel expenses and time, so look at the whole package to find what best meets your needs. For many, the chance to study with a particular master and the fact that they never have to take another Reiki class incline them to pay more for a situation that is particularly appealing. If there appears to be a financial barrier to studying with your preferred teacher, you can always open a discussion about options.

Look for a class that includes ample practice time, both for self-treatment and for sharing Reiki with the other students. If you practice enough in class, you'll feel comfortable continuing your practice at home. And remember, that's why you took the class—not just for the inspiring and rejuvenating experience of the class itself, not just to add another training to your résumé, but to be able to practice on your own forever after.

In the 1970s, Takata charged $125 for First Degree, $500 for Second Degree, and $10,000 for Reiki master training. Since her death in 1980, some masters have adjusted for inflation and charge more. Others have seen fit to charge less. First Degree classes today commonly cost between $100 and $500.

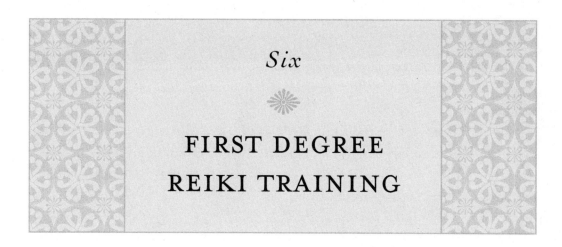

Six

FIRST DEGREE
REIKI TRAINING

Natural forces within us are the true healers of disease.

HIPPOCRATES

First Degree Reiki is where our practice begins. Once you've studied First Degree, you can simply place your hands gently on yourself or on someone else to offer healing. First Degree Reiki can be practiced by anyone who has the interest, regardless of the student's age or state of health. Although you will be taught specific hand placements to use (and I encourage you to use them), the most important thing for you to know is that at any given moment of need, you can access Reiki healing simply by placing your Reiki hand or hands on yourself or someone else, wherever you can. This is what First Degree training gives you.

I have seen many people with life-threatening illnesses surprised at how readily their First Degree–trained Reiki hands relieve aches and pains, restore clarity of mind, soften side effects of medications, and improve outlook. I've also seen healthy and hyper-functioning people come to see Reiki as an oasis: They can't relax on their own, but they're smart enough to read the writing on the wall. They know there's a reason health experts emphasize the importance of stress reduction to maintain optimal functioning, and they want to find the fastest, most reliable way possible to let off steam.

Most of the people I've trained in Reiki fall between these extremes, inhabiting every age, health, and socioeconomic bracket. I seek to instill in my students an enthusiasm for the practice, because when the class is over, it is the students' enthusiasm that supports them to continue practicing.

CHOOSING YOUR
FIRST DEGREE TEACHER

Once you've decided to learn to practice Reiki, the next step is to find a Reiki master. Please give this step the time and care it deserves. Your choice of Reiki master matters. The Reiki master who shares this practice with you will imprint your experience and understanding of Reiki. The Reiki master creates the setting and context for your learning. There is tremendous variety in the global Reiki menu. Some masters teach a practice encumbered by rules and regulations, unsound warnings, unnecessary complications, and false contraindications. Others give little or no instruction or support (offering initiations from the Internet, for example). You need to choose, from among all the options, the master and class situation that are right for you. This is an important decision, and chapter 5 addresses every aspect of it—locating masters in your area, identifying which ones meet your standards for credibility, and discovering which among those can best support you as you start your practice. Please consult chapter 5 before enrolling in a First Degree course. The litmus test for the choice you've made will be how inspired and enthusiastic you feel after the class, as you begin your practice.

THE CLASS

No two First Degree classes are alike. This is one of the things that make Reiki training so wonderful—but also difficult, in some ways, to describe. Although Takata organized the material very predictably over four successive sessions, she customized her presentation to each class. Even the most traditional Reiki masters I know don't teach exactly as Takata did, and rightly so. In order to serve as a steady and credible guide to one's students, a master must speak from his own experience and conviction. However, despite the variation in presentation, the material covered should be consistent.

As mentioned, First Degree Reiki training enables students to practice hands-on Reiki on themselves, rather than relying on a Reiki practitioner (professional or friend). In this training, students learn both abbreviated and full treatment protocols to be used when offering Reiki to themselves and to others. (You can also offer Reiki to your pets.)

Your Reiki master will give you an overview of Reiki history and present the Precepts Usui taught his students (which are discussed later in this chapter).

Most important, the class will include the initiations that empower students to practice. Takata gave four initiations to her First Degree students, one at a time, with ample time between each to absorb the benefit.

The basic structure of the class can and should be adapted to the students and circumstances, especially when teaching children, families, or the very ill. In most situations, approximately ten to twelve hours of class time are adequate to cover the basics, and allow for in-class practice time. Large classes may need more time. Students learn so much from one another that I hesitate to offer private training, except in special circumstances.

As of this writing, I most often teach First Degree in three four-hour classes spaced over a week. This format supports students in establishing their home practice, which is the point of learning Reiki. Students begin practicing in the first session. When they return to the second session, they share their experiences and ask the questions that come up only when you practice outside a class environment.

Don't expect to take notes in your Reiki class. Learning Reiki is not a scholarly pursuit. You may want to jot down some thoughts or points during breaks, or when you get home from class, but for the most part you want to rely on your practice rather than your mind to learn Reiki. Takata discouraged note-taking, saying "Just do it! Do Reiki, Reiki, Reiki, and then you shall know!"[1]

Some Reiki masters provide written materials for their students. Reiki classes taught in medical environments and accredited for continuing-education units (CEUs) or continuing medical education (CME) are required to include written materials.

For many, the First Degree training will be the only Reiki training they take, and all they will need. Even for those who continue to other levels of practice, what is learned in the First Degree training remains the foundation of Reiki practice.

INITIATION AND PRACTICE

Reiki training really doesn't teach us Reiki; it teaches us how to practice Reiki, and it is through practice, and practice alone, that we come to understand Reiki more deeply. And how do we practice? Takata was very clear: "First yourself."[2] Why is practice more important than study? Because Reiki is an empowered spiritual healing practice rather than a learned skill.

The empowerment to practice Reiki happens through the series of initiations shared by the Reiki master. An initiation is a concentrated sharing of Reiki that enables students to carry Reiki potential in their hands. Remember that Reiki is precipitated by the need of the person receiving treatment, whether the receiver is the practitioner or someone else. The initiation makes a connection through the biofield such that the healing pulsations originate not from the practitioner's own biofield, which would deplete him, but rather from the inexhaustible source that is accessed in the subtle heart. The transmission can be thought of as a subtle, gentle, yet powerful healing condensed into moments and subsequently developed through consistent practice. It is an open-ended process, a beginning with no end. The longer the student practices, the more Reiki and the student's understanding develop.

Students sometimes ask if something has been embedded in them during the initiations (a sure sign that a student has been reading). That's not my experience of initiation. Rather than adding something, I would say that the initiation process opens and strengthens what's already there, what is already ours: the access to primordial consciousness that is our birthright. The initiation creates an effortless and reliable link to the source of the pulsating consciousness we call Reiki.

IN-CLASS PRACTICE

In my First Degree classes, my students start practicing Reiki very early on, before there is too much discussion about what Reiki actually is. My intention is for students to learn to rely on their practice rather than their thoughts to understand Reiki from the very beginning. Too much talk puts the analytic mind in high gear as students struggle to understand something they have yet to experience. Why settle for theorizing when you can actually experience Reiki?

Many students come to learn Reiki having never received a Reiki treatment, but even those who have received treatment have yet to experience Reiki in their own hands. Bringing Reiki into our hands is a subtle and enormous empowerment, an experience that may seem beyond words. I encourage my students to simply be present to observe the opening created by the initiations. Once they begin practicing, students start to notice what is happening both in their hands and in their inner experience.

After each class practice session, I ask students to share their experiences, no matter how simple or subtle they might have been. It's always an interesting time—everyone has his own Reiki path. One person may experience peace, while another feels a cascade of bodily sensations, or a pleasant sense of fullness. There's often one student who sees colors or other visuals. Many students report hot hands. A cellist in one of my classes felt her hands had grown in size. A doctor inwardly saw her hands as made of light.

In 2004, I trained physicians as part of the Integrative Approaches to Depression medical conference in Tucson, Arizona. The class took place in a conference room in the hospital. As we were practicing, an emergency page came over the loudspeaker. Although none of my students were being paged, two of the doctors felt their Reiki hands activate, a dramatic demonstration of how unbalancing it is to be paged and of Reiki's rapid response to changes in our state of being.

Students don't always feel sensations right away. Instead, some notice a difference in how they feel *after* practicing. Other students don't think they felt anything, only recognizing their experience after hearing a classmate mention a similar sensation.

Each student benefits from revisiting his experience as he shares with the class, and everyone is introduced to the wide range of sensations and shifts that may accompany Reiki practice. I encourage each student to contribute to the discussion, even if all he has to say is, "I didn't notice anything." Admitting this aloud often takes the edge off the student's disappointment (or sense of failure) and gives me a chance to support him in his exploration. Sometimes, as students share, I may ask a question that helps them hone their observations and deepen their inner recognition.

Beginning students sometimes say, "I can't express what I'm feeling," or "I feel as if I went so far away that it's hard to go back there and remember," but I always encourage them to give it a shot. Expressing it—or even trying to—galvanizes the experience, validates it, and brings the inner into the outer world, where everything seems more real. People may have doubts about the "reality" of subtle inner experiences. (If you ever doubt that inner experiences are real, think about how easily you're affected by pain.)

If you are one who doesn't feel much (or anything) in the early practice sessions, don't worry. Just practice and allow Reiki to unfold naturally. Instead of feeling the soft pulsing associated with Reiki in your hands or body, you may notice the effect it has on you in other ways. You may feel calmer after practicing, or find you're sleeping better, waking earlier, and feeling more rested. One student of mine, a self-professed impatient driver, noticed he didn't run any red lights on his way to the second session. And enough students have ended lifelong constipation in their first class that part of my welcome speech includes the location of the plunger in the bathroom!

REIKI AND MEDITATION

Although it is not necessary to do so, I ask my students to meditate while I give the Reiki initiations and offer simple instructions to meditate on the breath. Meditation and Reiki are closely related. In fact, the very practice of Reiki arose out of Mikao Usui's meditation. I decided to learn to practice Reiki because within moments of a friend's placing hands on me for treatment, I felt the same subtle pulsations that I experienced in meditation. One reason I became a Reiki master was the recognition that for most people, Reiki is easier than meditation. And when the circumstances support it, Reiki practice often leads to a meditative state.

Part of everyone's developing relationship with Reiki is addressing skepticism and doubt. After all, we are used to working hard, our minds often working overtime, and Reiki is so simple. Some students need time to feel comfortable acknowledging an experience as simple and subtle as Reiki can be. Being in a meditative state can help. When the awareness is indrawn during the initiation, students are more likely to notice even a subtle shift in consciousness. Such an experience helps support them in the early days of practice, and often remains an inspiration many years later.

Another thing happens as we meditate in class: Students learn to observe their inner experiences without controlling or interpreting them. Meditation teaches us to detach from our thoughts and distractions. This is very useful when practicing Reiki, so that we can observe Reiki without making assumptions about our experience or jumping to false conclusions. Although Reiki experiences can be dramatic, they are often subtle. If we are able to connect our awareness with the subtlety, we will enjoy our practice more and we will practice more. And it's not that we *have* to observe Reiki—Reiki does what it does whether we are watching or not—but observing Reiki during some of your practice time will deepen your understanding and motivate you to continue practicing.

TREATMENT PROTOCOLS

First Degree students learn a basic protocol for treatment that traditionally consists of a series of eight or nine hand placements for self-treatment and an additional four placements on the back when treating others. As with all aspects of Reiki practice, there is considerable variation among different practitioners, with some common threads. Treatment typically starts at the head and continues downward to the lower abdomen. Consistent with Asian medicine, the hand placements are on the head and torso over the endocrine glands and organs that control overall function and well-being. Using the full protocol guarantees that the essential areas that govern well-being are refreshed, so that the underlying imbalance is addressed.

Using the full protocol also means that beginning students can be confident they are giving a complete treatment even if they don't yet feel secure following the pulsations in their hands. We simplify our practice by using a habitual sequence when giving treatment, but it can be just as effective and not in any way dangerous to place hands out of sequence, or to start somewhere other than the head. Sometimes Takata said to start treatment with the head. Other times she said the abdomen. Sometimes she said it didn't matter where the treatment started as long as students used the full protocol. Although she stressed using all the hand placements she taught, Takata did not want her students to be rigid in their practice. She encouraged students to develop their intuitive feel for treatment while being mindful of the full series of hand placements. Takata said, "Reiki will guide you. Let the Reiki hands find it. They will know what to do."[3] While Takata taught her students to honor the body as a whole by using the full protocol, she also encouraged placing Reiki hands right where it hurt.

Some practitioners prefer to place a folded tissue over the eyes of the person being treated. When touching another person, we want to be particularly gentle around the face and the throat. If she was sure that the person wasn't wearing contact lenses, Takata would put light pressure on the eyelids. I prefer to cup my hands over the eyes and the larynx (some people will involuntarily gag if the front of their throat is touched). Place hands carefully at the lower abdomen and on a woman's upper chest so as not to be invasive.

PRECEPTS

Most of life happens when we're not practicing Reiki. How can we create a container to hold the benefits of Reiki so they filter down into our daily lives? Usui offered his students precepts to support their practice, guidelines to engage their awareness and protect them in moments of uncertainty. Like wise words from all great traditions, the precepts are timeless and transcultural, as relevant today as they were in early-twentieth-century Japan.

The precepts are traditionally presented in First Degree training, where they create a strong support for your practice of Reiki. They become increasingly meaningful as your practice matures. Usui advised his students to repeat the precepts every morning and evening and considered them part of the practice. I particularly encourage students who don't have another spiritual practice to use the precepts as tools to engage the mind in maintaining balance, a compass to guide choices and actions. They're not additional commandments, nor are they a list of "shoulds." They are simply contemplations to inform our choices.

Here are the precepts as Takata presented them to her students:[4]

Just for today, do not worry.
Just for today, do not anger.
Honor your parents, teachers, and elders.
Earn your living honestly.
Show gratitude to every living thing.

There are various translations of the precepts floating around. Knowing that Japanese is a contextual language, organized completely differently from English, I was never satisfied by assurances that "this is the exact translation." I asked a Japanese student of mine, a man in a position of responsibility at the United Nations, to help. I gave Toshi a copy of the precepts in Japanese and various translations I had gathered. His response surprised me. Whereas translations invariably list five precepts, Toshi assured me there are really four. What are usually translated in English as the third and fourth precepts are written in Japanese as one, connected by a conjunction indicating that the second part builds on the first. The two parts formulate one concept. Furthermore, I was told, there are no words such as *ancestors, parents,* or *elders* in the third precept, and the word *gratitude* does not appear in the last precept. I confirmed this with other people fluent in Japanese. Through e-mail, I discussed this with Hyakuten Inamoto, a Japanese Buddhist monk and Reiki master initiated by Hayashi's student, Chiyoko Yamaguchi. He concurred and offered his translation of the precepts:

Today only
Do not anger
Do not worry
With thankfulness
Work diligently
Be kind to others

We Americans pride ourselves on being pragmatic and explicit. We like things spelled out for us. "Give it to me straight," we say.

Other cultures don't hold this value of plain talk. One of the greatest differences between Japanese culture and language and American culture and language lies in the area of implicit/explicit. It is not a Japanese expectation that expression be simple and straightforward. Subtlety and nuance are prized. What is *not* said in Japanese is expressed as much as what *is* said. A student of mine who is first-generation Japanese-American has spoken of the difficulties Japanese people have communicating with her generation. There is so much that is expected to be understood, and when one is raised in another country, it's not. Translating from Japanese to American isn't a matter of translating words as much as translating a culture and its values. We cannot be literal without missing the point. (Our respect for Takata's accomplishment in bringing Reiki to America grows the more we understand this.)

In an attempt to bridge this cultural gap, and with respect for the Japanese preference for odd-numbered groupings, here are the precepts as I have rendered them:

> *Just for today, do not be angry and do not worry.*
> *Value your life and make the effort necessary to actualize your life's purpose.*
> *Be kind.*

The precepts start with the reminder *Just for today.* This phrase signifies the present, right now, this moment. This is the moment that is ours. If we think forever, we get lost, but eternity is simply the eternal present. Staying in the present, staying present, makes everything else possible.

My colleague Kumiko Kanayama is an accomplished practitioner of Ohashiatsu® and Reiki, who moved to New York City from Hiroshima in 1987. She explains, "Chronological time is different from west and east. Just for today means forever, just for today means only today. It is hard to explain but life is a circle, it comes and goes."

The precepts provide a compass we can use to adjust our inner behavior, our state, what we do before we take outer action. For example, if I don't know what to do about a situation that has angered me, the precepts remind me to address my anger first. If I'm worrying about something and frustrated that there's nothing I can do about it, the precepts point me toward what I *can* do, which is to address my worried state, because worry is negative prayer. The precepts don't mean that one never fights; rather, one never fights from anger. The precepts protect us. After all, *we* suffer the most from the negativity we hold in our minds.

Just for today, do not be angry and do not worry does not mean one should engage in blind faith or adopt a passive God-will-take-care-of-it attitude. Life brings the necessity to act, and we each have the opportunity to take right action. True spirituality has teeth. Even those who advocate radical nonviolence are not feckless pushovers. The state of mind from which we take action affects the outcome, so the spiritual practitioner cultivates evenness of temperament. This is not to be mistaken for a flattening of affect or an inability to feel, an inauthentic spiritual bypass out of the present, but rather the ability to feel emotions while witnessing them without attachment. (For those who would like to explore this further, Gurumayi Chidvilasananda's book *Courage and Contentment* offers both insight and practical guidance on how to anchor ourselves in steadiness, which can be an inspiring companion as we explore living with the precepts.)

Reiki offers the experience of connectedness, and the precepts remind us of that connectedness so that our actions are aligned with our true being and the benefit of all. *Just for today, do not be angry and do not worry* cautions us to address negative emotions early, before they lead to misguided behavior. Feeling disconnected and powerless gives rise to anger and anxiety. Once we restore the sense of connectedness, we feel good about our lives and are motivated to express our gifts. Aware of our connectedness, we naturally express kindness. This understanding of interconnectedness is common in indigenous cultures in various parts of the world. It was a living priority in the lives of pre-Columbian native Americans, expressed to this day by the phrase *All my relations.*[5] In Africa, it is said, "I am because we are."[6]

The combined third and fourth precepts, *Be thankful and work diligently,* or *Value your life and make the effort necessary to actualize your life's purpose,* express the concept of dharma that is valued throughout Asian spirituality. Each of us is born with a specific nature, temperament, constitution (ask any mother who has given birth to more than one child). Our greatest gift to the world is to develop ourselves and express our uniqueness. *Dharma* is often translated as "righteousness," but the moralistic tone of this word is misleading. Dharma is refining the natural expression of our inherent goodness through our unique nature.

Each of us has something unique and valuable to offer, and it's not separate from who we are. It is not simply that we have a talent; it's the whole package that the talent comes wrapped in—our individuality. But we don't want to offer it to the world half-baked. Effort is needed to polish our understanding and our gifts, the effort of self-discovery and honing our tools. The point is not to pursue becoming something we are not, but rather to take the steps needed to mature, to be more authentically who we are, and to learn the skills needed to express our gifts in the world. The effort needed is largely discipline (for example, as related to the precepts) and spiritual practices such as meditation, contemplation, and self-inquiry.

Lest anyone think this concept is irrelevant foreign philosophy, I offer a quote from modern-dance pioneer Martha Graham.

> There is a vitality, a life force, an energy, a quickening, that is translated through you into action, and because there is only one of you in all time, this expression is unique. And if you block it, it will never exist through any other medium and will be lost. It is your sole responsibility to keep the channel open.

In Takata's rendition of the precepts, *Honor our parents, teachers and elders* and *Earn your living honestly* succinctly and pragmatically express dharmic action in contemporary everyday life in a way that was particularly relevant and accessible to her audience. Traditionally, honoring the ancestors helped one find oneself in the larger context of what has come before. And in a less mobile society, the work by which one earns a living is also one's offering to the community.

The essence of *Show gratitude to every living thing* is distilled in the simple phrase *Be kind.* Gratitude begets kindness. The word translated as "kind" in Japanese also implies sincerity. According to either translation, the final precept echoes the sense of authenticity encouraged by *With thankfulness, work diligently.* The process is not a matter of overcoming our true nature, but rather of removing obstacles so that the authentic self can shine. It is an affirmation of our inherent beneficence, the unifield field, primordial consciousness, Reiki.

There is much overlap between these precepts and other guides to right living. Timeless virtues such as equanimity, self-restraint, gratitude, right effort, and kindness are respected cross-culturally. For example, *ahimsa,* the yogic injunction against violence, could be understood to proscribe anger and worry and promote right effort and gratitude, which in turn begets respect and kindness. It is expressed in conventional medicine in the Hippocratic Oath: *First do no harm.*

The precepts are ongoing contemplations on living. Choose the translation that most appeals to you, the one that you remember easily. It's valuable to have the precepts as available to your awareness as Reiki is to your hand.

DAILY SELF-TREATMENT

Give yourself a full treatment each day (perhaps more often if you are ill) and experiment with moments of Reiki throughout your day, finding times when your hands are not busy doing other things. If my students are any indication, a lot of Reiki is done in New York City buses and subways, and in the backs of cabs. Of course in public settings, it's wise to place Reiki hands discreetly.

One of Reiki's great advantages is that it can be practiced, surreptitiously if necessary, in any setting: during a meeting that is either stressful or just plain boring, while waiting in line at the bank, or even when watching TV. One of my HIV+ students came to appreciate Reiki after placing hands for treatment while watching a few hours of TV in the evening. When he shut off the tube to go to bed, he noticed that he felt really good—centered, balanced, and pain-free. He knew TV had never made him feel like that before and realized it must be Reiki.

It's reassuring to know that Reiki hands are available and responsive whenever needed, since emergencies and daily dramas don't schedule themselves to our convenience. At times of greater or lesser trauma, we can always place a Reiki hand anywhere and experience its balancing effect, even while calling 911. Medics attest that it's easier to treat a calm patient than one who is disoriented by pain and fear.

Although placing Reiki hands anywhere anytime will bring benefit, there is no question that the best results come with consistent daily practice of the full protocol over a period of time. I ask students to commit to practicing at least six months before evaluating the difference Reiki can make in their lives. My hope is that by then they will have transitioned from the honeymoon afterglow of class into enthusiastic commitment to their daily practice.

The more we practice, the greater our understanding and the greater our understanding, the more committed we are to practice. It's that simple. We learn how to practice in class and our continued practice reveals Reiki to us gradually over time. Reiki is almost technique-less, so there's no reason to worry. You can't do Reiki wrong. You can, however, do it without understanding or respect for the process. That's not wrong, but it's less gratifying.

To get the most from your First Degree training, I encourage you to create your Reiki routine and practice regularly. If you do, your daily practice will pay dividends on your Reiki investment for life. Over more than two decades of practicing and eighteen years of teaching, I've probably addressed every possible obstacle to daily practice in either myself or my students. Here are some tips to support your practice.

Daily Practice Logistics

It's easiest to practice regularly if you locate a place in your life for Reiki. This is easily accomplished because, unlike meditation, Reiki can be practiced in short spurts or even, if need be, while doing something else. Make two choices to create a foundation for your daily practice to rest on, and it will quickly become a daily haven. Decide where and when—where in your home is your favorite Reiki spot and when in your daily routine will you be in that place to practice?

The answer for many people is their bed either in the morning or at night, or both. Most students find practicing Reiki in bed as they awaken or fall asleep brings the benefits of daily practice without putting any strain on their busy schedules. It's not uncommon for students who practice in the morning to start awakening to find their hands are already in place. And what could be easier than giving yourself Reiki as you fall asleep? Even if you don't finish your routine, Reiki continues to flow as long as it's needed, and you can pick up where you left off the next night.

Of course you can also find other times to practice. One psychotherapist I trained gives herself Reiki during the late-afternoon break between her day and evening patients.

Busy moms might take a few minutes for Reiki curled up on the sofa after getting the family off on weekday mornings, and have alternate weekend routines. Find the place and time that is easiest for you.

Daily Practice: Finding the Motivation

When you first learn Reiki, it will be easy to practice regularly. The experience is new and pleasurable and fascinating and flexible. With continued practice over time, however, the experience will become more subtle, less dramatic. Students sometimes fear this means their Reiki is weakening. This is one of many false judgments that can wreak havoc with our practice. Actually it's a *good* sign when Reiki becomes quieter, evidence that the balancing needed is on subtler rather than grosser levels of our being. This is an indication of health.

When we start our practice, there's usually a bit of a shift needed to bring us toward balance. Reiki is busy balancing our biofield and beyond, precipitating adjustments on mental, emotional, and physical levels, and our sessions reflect this activity. When we've practiced regularly for a while, we live closer to center and, unless something dramatic is happening in our lives or we get run down, there's not so much obvious rearranging to be done. This is a critical point in your practice. Don't get discouraged and fall out of the habit just because it's not so apparently powerful. In fact, your treatment at this time may be *more* powerful, and the prevention you accomplish through daily practice is immeasurable. Any day that you miss your practice, not only are you missing the sweet, centered feeling Reiki imparts, but you're also missing an opportunity to nip future imbalances in the bud.

Commit yourself to practicing at a certain point in your day, every day, and you will never stray farther than twenty-four hours from your center. On days that are unusually packed, you can always do an abbreviated treatment, but be sure to return to your full treatment the next day.

Musicians and athletes value practice, and that's a good start, but spiritual practice is a little different. We're not looking to improve performance but rather to deepen our understanding. There is a depth that comes only with continued practice over time, that arises both from the benefits the practice itself brings and from the friction created by our interface with the discipline of daily practice, how we tame ourselves through daily practice. We can be disciplined without being rigid. We can be disciplined and be gentle and kind with ourselves.

Beware of another practice pitfall: perfectionism. Don't let perfectionism keep you from practicing. Remember, you can't make a mistake with Reiki. If it seems too much to do a full treatment, start with a modified treatment for the first week or so. Choose your favorite placement on your head, then place hands on your chest and your abdomen. When you're ready, you can simply add another placement one at a time. Take as long as you like to increase to the eight basic placements.

Although at first it may seem like a big deal to give yourself treatment, soon it will be as easy as fluffing the duvet to freshen your bed. Be light with your practice. Enjoy it. Remember Takata's encouragement: "Some Reiki is better than none at all."

WILL READING SUPPORT MY PRACTICE?

Students often ask, "What can I read?" I appreciate their enthusiasm to learn more about Reiki, and I've created a website, www.ReikiInMedicine.org, and authored medical papers, popular articles, and now a book to help. However, once they start practicing First Degree, I encourage my students to put the reading material aside until they are comfortably established in their practice.

Reading can inform us about Reiki, but we don't learn Reiki through reading. We learn Reiki through practice. If you wanted to learn painting, you would get only so far by reading books on painting, wouldn't you? At some point, you would have to surrender to the actual act of painting. The same is true of Reiki. I hope you will think of this book as your lifelong Reiki companion, but also keep time simply to be alone with Reiki and let your Reiki hands teach you.

If you've perused the existing Reiki literature, you know what a broad range of practice styles is represented. Facing contradictory information or speaking with a friend who was trained differently too early in your practice can be confusing and disheartening.

I recommend giving yourself time simply to practice in the way you were trained. As your practice progresses and deepens, there may come a time when you find it stimulating to explore other approaches, but don't let your head get in the way of your hands.

AFTER THE CLASS: TAKING REIKI HOME

Transition from class to home by placing your Reiki hands on your body as soon as you can after class is over. Let moments of spot treatment scattered through your day be stepping-stones to carry you between your full treatments.

What may take some getting used to is never knowing when Reiki will kick in or what Reiki will do. A First Degree student once reached across the bed for her husband as she awoke on the day after her first class, resting her hand on his shoulder to say good morning. Moments later, he asked, "What's going on in your hand?" You may unexpectedly feel Reiki in your hand as you stroke your cat or dog.

Sometimes as I am demonstrating hand placements on a student in class, Reiki will whoosh forth as soon as I place my hands on my "dummy." Physicians and other hands-on health-care providers notice Reiki pulsing sometimes during the brief touch of a medical exam or physical therapy. Occasionally a handshake will activate my palms.

Students notice different effects from their new Reiki practice. Some changes are obvious, but healing also shows up in unexpected ways. Speaking to one of my first students a few months after her First Degree training, I learned that although she enjoyed the practice, she hadn't noticed any benefits coming from it. But oh, by the way, she had finally learned to drive a car (at age forty), gotten her driver's license, driven to her country house alone for the first time, and spent the night there by herself—also a first. Add to all that the detail of how her husband had wanted to mortgage the country house—the only property in the marriage that was hers alone—and she negotiated an arrangement with him that proved very advantageous when they divorced not long afterward. After hearing all this, I laughed aloud. "And you think nothing has come of your Reiki practice?" I asked incredulously. She laughed, too. What hadn't occurred to her before was now very obvious.

Another student came to learn Reiki as part of a career change. He was a casualty of the dot-com bust in his midthirties and struggling to redirect his life. Although his wife's successful law practice provided a buffer against financial pressures, being dependent upon her salary taxed his already challenged self-esteem. He'd grown sullen and snappish and feared his future was melting like chocolate in the sun. Not knowing much about Reiki but thinking he might pursue a career in alternative health care, he signed up for my First Degree class. This affable man presented as a disoriented computer geek with no life experience to prepare him for the change Reiki brought. What amazed him even more than the improvements in sleep, anxiety, confidence, and motivation was the feedback from his friends and family, who were delighted that their beleaguered friend had gone to the coast for a "business conference" and come back his old self.

To get your Reiki practice off to a strong start:

1. Practice Reiki on yourself every day.
2. Choose a time and place and "just do it."
3. Give yourself a full treatment whenever possible, but be flexible. If a placement seems particularly active and you want to let your hands linger there, do so; what you don't finish at one session you can pick up again later or tomorrow.
4. Become immersed in daily hands-on Reiki (usually a minimum of three months) before taking Second Degree training.
5. Remember, hands-on self-treatment remains the foundation of Reiki at all levels of practice.

Seven

※

SECOND DEGREE
REIKI TRAINING

What is here, is also there; what is not here, is nowhere.

VISHVASARA TANTRA, KATHA UPANISHAD

Second Degree Reiki training enables students to offer Reiki to others without touch, moving Reiki practice into the more nebulous realm of distant, non-touch healing. "More nebulous" does not mean less real and it certainly doesn't mean less effective, but the idea of distant healing can incite the inner skeptic to new levels of protest. Perhaps the reality that Reiki is not "figure-outable" is never as apparent as when giving distant healing treatments. Yet distant healing can be seen as simply a nonreligious form of prayer, and prayer specifically for health is by far the "complementary and alternative therapy" most commonly used in America.[1]

Why would you want to learn to offer Reiki without touching? Many people are content with the hands-on practice they learn in First Degree training, and I rarely encourage students to learn Second Degree. There is no need to take more Reiki training when you can deepen your practice ad infinitum simply by practicing hands-on regularly.

There are, however, some practical reasons for learning Second Degree. Professionals, such as psychiatrists, psychotherapists, guidance counselors, and teachers may want to bring healing into their work, but touch is not within their scope of practice. Others seek Second Degree training to empower their own spiritual practices. Some students have family members living elsewhere who would like to receive distant healing. And then there are students who simply love Reiki, practice regularly, and want to expand their Reiki horizons. All these are valid reasons for continuing your Reiki training. It's just important not to assume that "more is better."

Unless there is a good reason to move more quickly (which I occasionally encounter), I encourage students to practice hands-on Reiki for three to six months before enrolling in a Second Degree class. I have never seen a student lose through waiting, but I have seen many students who literally lost touch with their practice because they moved too fast. I don't see any benefit for students who aren't practicing regularly to learn distant treatment, so I only accept students who are practicing daily self-treatment into a Second Degree class. Without daily hands-on self-treatment, there is no foundation on which to build distant healing. Second Degree is not another tool to add to one's healing kit; it's a practice.

When I meet people who have been trained in Reiki, but who are not practicing, I find that almost invariably they have taken First and Second Degree training (and sometimes more) very close together, often in the same weekend. Taking that many initiations in such a short period of time does not allow much chance for digestion. Condensed training also does not give students much practice time, and students who don't feel confident in what they are doing are less likely to continue practicing. If students are taught by a traveling Reiki master who doesn't offer ongoing support, it's easy to see how daily practice can wind up as roadkill on the busy highway of contemporary lifestyle.

WHAT IS SECOND DEGREE PRACTICE?

In Second Degree training, students learn how to replace the hand-to-body connection with the mind, using three symbols that have been passed from Reiki master to

Reiki master-in-training since Mikao Usui. Because students need to learn both the symbols and how and when to use them, there is considerably more technical learning in the Second Degree class than in First Degree. However, with attention and disciplined practice, students become so fluent in Second Degree technique that it is no more cumbersome than hands-on First Degree class practice. Additionally, Second Degree precipitates a deepening and strengthening of the student's access to Reiki.

As in the First Degree class, you'll practice your new skills on yourself and the other students. You'll also practice distant healing sessions and receive an initiation to establish your connection with the symbols discussed in the next few pages.

Like First Degree Reiki, Second Degree technique can be applied in a variety of ways. You can use the Second Degree symbols for brief or full distant sessions when treating yourself or when treating other people. The symbols can also enhance either spot or full hands-on treatment. Just as in First Degree self-treatment, you can offer distant Reiki even when you're preoccupied with other things.

Second Degree students have experiences and notice changes in themselves from the very first class, just as they did in First Degree. Because Reiki helps heal deeply rooted systemic imbalances, students' responses to learning Second Degree are often, but not necessarily, an expanded echo of their First Degree benefits. A student who felt more grounded when she started practicing Reiki will likely feel even more grounded in the Second Degree class. A student who noticed a surge in motivation and productivity with First Degree may well feel another with Second Degree.

An artist in her late twenties reported feeling less tired and more confident. She went to a social event attended by high-powered professionals in her field and was surprised at how comfortable she felt in a setting she previously found intimidating. She also felt steadier, not so easily knocked off center by strong emotions. Other students report different benefits, such as experiencing greater intimacy, feeling more decisive or more empowered, feeling kinder and more empathic, or simply feeling more like themselves and liking themselves more, feeling more in control of their lives, and more accepting of the parts they can't control.

NOW DO I HAVE TO "BELIEVE"?

Reiki is never a matter of belief; it is a path of practice. Students who have significant experience with subtle realities before learning Second Degree, either through months or more of daily hands-on practice or, as in my case, years of meditation, have a significant advantage over those who don't. Following this path of practice eases the mind gently past the inner skeptic, which may squeak and protest from time to time, but which comes to realize it has no case to argue in the court of examined experience. When a practitioner already has the conviction, born of practice, that Reiki can heal through light touch, replacing touch with a mental procedure is not such a leap as it is for one who has no prior experience with vibrational reality. In order for the student to fully appreciate what Reiki practice can bring, especially during a crisis or when someone is unconscious, it is important that Reiki remain a matter of experience and not become a matter of belief.

Unlike magic or shamanistic practices, the power of Reiki is not wielded by the practitioner. The practitioner merely carries Reiki potential, which activates spontaneously in response to need. Reiki is not controlled or manipulated in any way by a practitioner at any level of experience or training. Since Reiki does not originate in the mind, it is not mind over matter, nor is it mind/body medicine. This is a tenet that remains constant throughout all levels of Reiki training.

DISTANT HEALING

Distant healing is an even greater affront to the skeptical mind than first experiencing Reiki in your own hands. Whenever possible, I have people who want to receive distant treatment during the class on standby. Getting quick feedback builds students' confidence. When it's time to practice in class, I call the person who wants healing and suggest she lie down alone in a room to rest. I ask her to call me in fifteen minutes if she is awake (I don't want her to set an alarm) or else e-mail in the morning. Since most of my classes are in the evening, the chances of the receiver's falling asleep for the best night's sleep she's had in a while are pretty high, but when someone is awake to share her experience of receiving, it greatly supports the learning process.

One of my volunteers, a breast-cancer patient, was still experiencing postsurgical pain, especially under her left arm. Her experience of chemotherapy had been particularly grueling. That and a bout of pneumonia left her exhausted, and she was about to start radiation. While my Second Degree students practiced by sending her a distant healing, she experienced an overall sense of comfort, suffused by what she described as a warm soothing feeling. She felt a warm tingling where she had had pain and slept particularly well that night.

Once we move out of the touch mode of practice, it doesn't matter how near or far we are from the person to whom we are sending treatment. Reiki is not like a radio that can be out of range. It's the omnipresent, dimensionless, unified field in which everything exists. Across the room or across the sea, it's all within reach of distant healing.

Takata taught Second Degree in a completely straightforward manner. Takata's student Reiki master Paul David Mitchell explains, "With Mrs. Takata, it was understood that offering a distant treatment implied that you had a Reiki relationship with that person." Mitchell remembers the story of a student asking Takata if one needed permission to send a distant treatment. Takata replied quizzically, "Why would you want to send a treatment to someone who didn't want it?"

SECOND DEGREE SYMBOLS

First Degree practice is so simple; everything we need is in our hands. Second Degree practice is different. In your Second Degree class, you will learn three Reiki symbols, or *kotodama*. The symbols are profound images that connect us to primordial consciousness.[2] The Second Degree initiation opens and establishes our relationship with these symbols, and our continuing practice sustains that relationship. We use the symbols to create the connection through which Reiki healing can activate. They are used for distant healing when we are unable to touch, or to enhance the hand-to-body connection. When you first meet the Reiki symbols, it can seem like a lot of information. Don't worry; just practice. Proficiency and ease will come with practice, and sooner than you think.

There is much difference of opinion in today's diverse Reiki community regarding the Second Degree symbols. Traditionally, the symbols are shared only with those who have taken the Second Degree initiation. According to Hiroshi Doi, a Japanese Reiki master and member of the Gakkai, this has been a pragmatic restriction, since no one outside the community of trained students would know what to do with the symbols.[3] The traditional Takata-based community has maintained this discipline of privacy, sometimes enshrouding the symbols with a devotional air.

The rapid proliferation of Reiki since the late 1980s spread Reiki techniques much faster than it spread Reiki understanding. Once people who had little or no practical Reiki experience were initiated as masters, the traditions of Reiki seemed out of date, and to some people, keeping "secrets" seemed downright un-American rather than a matter of practicality or respect. Although it is understandable how this happened, traditions exist to convey the deepest meaning and value of a practice, to carry the context in which practice is meaningful. When we honor traditions and we practice diligently, we protect the profound aspects of Reiki and guarantee that they will be available to coming generations. When we overlook traditions, we lose the benefit of their guidance and protection. As Reiki was spread indiscriminately through American and western European countries, cultures not embedded with Asian spiritual practices, the value of tradition was not communicated and the traditions were often lost.

WHY THE SECRECY?

Although many Founding Fathers belonged to the secret Order of Freemasons, Americans today are suspicious of secrecy. We view it not as respect or deference or discretion or any of the mature connotations it can carry, but rather as a sign of elitism or an affront to the great American values of freedom and equality. In the context of

Reiki, this is simply not the case. Reiki originated in a culture rich with deference and decorum, one in which the implicit is equally important as the explicit, or perhaps even more important. Additionally, whereas American culture venerates intrepid pioneers, Japanese culture frowns on treading where one does not belong.

Having given his students the initial teachings, Usui gave them more advanced teachings according to how diligently they practiced and what they attained through practice. Usui did not give advanced teachings to novices. This is common in Asian spirituality.

Advanced practices are usually kept private, for many reasons. One reason is simply a sense of appropriateness and respect. Another is to protect the power of the practice. *The Buddhist Handbook* explains that some practices are traditionally kept restricted because "malpractice weakens their effectiveness: the spiritual equivalent of debasing the coinage."[4]

Such a traditional perspective may not seem relevant to contemporary students, but it is protective of the student as well as the practice. Keeping the secrecy of the symbols helps to maintain the process as an inner process, so we don't fall prey to outer distractions, and so we don't wander unknowingly into magical thinking, which can easily happen in the boundaryless realm of distant healing. Secrecy can also be a way to keep the symbols as tools that are meaningful to a very specific scope of practice.

SECOND DEGREE IN DAILY PRACTICE

Daily practice takes on another level of importance once you start using Second Degree. When first introduced to the symbols, there is always a student who turns to me wide-eyed and asks, "How can I ever remember them?" It makes me smile. I remember my Second Degree class very well. I remember the first time I saw each symbol, the inner response I noticed, and the intuitive understanding that blossomed as I contemplated the image. I also remember thinking, *Am I* really *supposed to be able to learn this?* But in no time, Second Degree became second nature. Now I remember the symbols the same way I remember the phone number my family had when I was a kid—repeated, daily use. I use the Reiki symbols every day, many times a day, in addition to my hands-on practice. How else could I possibly remember them?

By the time I learned to practice Reiki, I was already a professional healer using a spectrum of mind/body techniques to enhance awareness and alignment and promote healing. I didn't need any encouragement to start exploring uses of Second Degree Reiki beyond sending treatment to a particular person. The possible uses of Second Degree practice are unlimited. It can be used to offer Reiki to groups of people—a family or a surgical team—or to encourage balance in relationships or situations.

Reiki is unlimited and omnipresent. Released from the linearity of hand-to-body contact, the Second Degree practitioner can reach beyond physical limitations, including time and space. But while Reiki is unlimited, the practitioner's understanding of it may not be. If you are going to explore the possible uses of distant treatment, I urge you to stay mindful of your own experience.

First of all, do you feel anything? Second Degree students often feel their hands activate when giving distant treatment in a way similar to when they touch. Second, be mindful that you are not trying to manipulate anyone or anything: Reiki will not bend to your will. Rather, think of Second Degree treatment as sending a fortunate blessing to uplift the entire situation and everyone involved. Don't let this become a power trip, a fantasy, or a delusion. Stay with what is real to you. Play the tension between the concept of what is possible and what you actually experience, and restrict yourself to those applications that are personally meaningful.

As with First Degree practice, how you practice is not important (within reason); *that* you practice, and practice daily, is. Let your practice be guided by your experience, not by your mind. Otherwise it will become very abstract and lose its sweetness and you will fall away from it. Don't get theoretical; keep it visceral. One day you may feel very expanded and experience something that can seem rather tenuous on another day. Stay present for each day's practice *as it is*.

At the same time, I encourage you to contemplate your experiences. A contemplated practice is a richer practice. You know how a movie replays in the mind for a while afterward, even showing up in dreams that night? Why not use contemplation to similarly lengthen our Reiki experiences, allowing them to ripen into insight?

PRACTICE GUIDANCE

It may not be wise to practice Second Degree on your family members until you are confident of your technique, because the emotional attachments to family members can confuse or clutter the experience. Practice first on the people to whom your teacher has arranged for you to send treatment. Not knowing them personally will keep the experience clear and build your confidence. Students often end these class practice sessions glowing. They are surprised by the sense of intimacy felt when sending distant treatment to people they don't know. This is what happens when we dip into the unified field: We as well as those to whom we offer healing are uplifted. At all levels of practice, Reiki heals the practitioner as well as the recipient.

Whenever you doubt if it's okay to offer distant healing to someone else, offer yourself Reiki instead. It's very human to want to heal the people we love, and it's easy to trespass boundaries by trying to heal what we haven't been asked to heal (and what may actually be our problem rather than our loved one's). If we treat ourselves instead, we may be able to heal the fear in us that makes us overprotective, perhaps to the point of being controlling or even judgmental of those we love. It is safest to offer Reiki from a place of trust, not because Reiki is ever dangerous, but because our minds can be. But in moments when we can't trust, we can still safely offer ourselves Reiki. Become comfortable with your practice of Second Degree Reiki and experience profoundly your direct relationship with Reiki.

USES OF DISTANT HEALING

Distant healing can work in unexpected ways. A friend called asking for treatment one morning as I was getting my young children ready for school. I agreed, but the request got lost in my hectic morning, and I didn't remember to send the treatment until four in the afternoon. The next day, when she called to thank me, she mentioned that although usually she would feel better soon after calling me, this time things didn't shift until after four that afternoon. Other times I've spoken to clients on the phone and felt Reiki mobilizing so rapidly—without my setting up the distant protocols—that I told my clients to go rest and call back later if they still felt they needed something. Those calls were never made.

Once we are no longer restricted to offering Reiki to that which we can touch, the applications of Reiki are limited only by our concepts. Anything can be supported to move toward harmony. Reiki healing strikes a note of commonality, switching attention from what separates us to what we have in common. It's very much the way I experience my hands when giving treatment, as if they were vibrating with the unique sound of my client's well-being, bringing remembered wellness into the forefront of his attention.

The same healing process that happens at the level of a single human being can be offered to group endeavors—meetings or classes, for example, or the list of people requesting healing prayers at your place of worship (unless you don't think Reiki qualifies as "healing prayer"). This healing process can be applied to anything, even politics—not to make others agree with our values but to support the functioning of our democratic process. Imagine blue- and red-state Reiki practitioners offering distant treatment to the White House and/or Congress. (That gives a whole new meaning to bipartisanship!) Or perhaps there is a cause that you support, such as the effort to end global warming or world hunger. It's up to you. Just remember that Reiki supports balance, that you cannot use Reiki to manipulate a specific result.

Second Degree Reiki practice frees us from the inherent boundaries of touch. You might land in a wide-open field of targets in need of healing, and drive yourself nuts treating everyone who crosses your mind in a day and every dire situation in the headlines. When your head is spinning with the possibilities, remember freedom is self-control. And how can we control ourselves before we go spiraling off into assuming responsibility to heal the world one detail at a time? Remember that the foundation of Reiki practice is self-healing. While you're practicing self-treatment, check up, meaning perform self-inquiry, and examine your motivations. Are you offering Reiki from a contented mind or are you driven by a vague, discomforting sense of guilt to fix the universe? While coupling self-treatment and contemplation in this way, we might be drawn into a profound awareness that we make our greatest offering to the world simply by attending to our own balance. Every time we create peace in our own being, we make a significant contribution to world peace.

Here are some of the ways in which I have applied Second Degree Reiki with good results. Some students pick up on these applications and others don't, or there may be one particular application that you find appealing.

Stressful Situations

We have all found ourselves knee-deep in difficulties involving circumstances or other people that made us want to throw our hands up and run away. On the way to resolution, we may have to say or hear things that evoke strong emotion and fear. Reiki can help. Send a distant treatment to the situation. If there are meetings or confrontations, use the symbols before, during, and after, if you feel shaken or unresolved. Reiki can relieve hostility and enhance our capacity for understanding, enabling us to hear another's perspective without defensiveness. It can also help those who would be victimized rise to their own clear and reasonable defense, supporting them to set rational and healthy boundaries without blaming or provoking others.

Problem Solving

One morning, with my students due to arrive for a Second Degree class, one of the bathrooms started flooding. I know nothing about plumbing, especially plumbing that's nearly one hundred years old. As I instinctively began offering Reiki to the situation, my eye was drawn to a particular valve. I turned it, and the water stopped. This is a good example of how Reiki can support balance practically in situations as well as in humans.

A hard-line skeptic might say if Reiki was real, the water would have stopped flooding on its own. Maybe I'm "Reiki lite," but it seems that magical thinking isn't useful in most people's lives. Having access to healing consciousness doesn't keep us from having to take action. Taking a second to create alignment through Reiki can keep us from flailing our arms in anxious confusion and guide us to make the effort that will bring results. As we enhance alignment through Reiki, it's easier to identify where the adjustments need to be made, and then to take appropriate action.

Relationships

While we can send distant healing to support balance in any relationship, we may be tempted at times to send a distant treatment to "heal" our friend or spouse into seeing things our way. But this isn't how Reiki works. Reiki will not manipulate the person you're struggling with to see your perspective but may, instead, open you to understand his. Reiki brings balance. If a relationship has become snagged and you're willing to see your role in it, try a distant-healing session for the relationship itself. You may immediately sense an opening, or your experience of the session may be unremarkable and things may start moving later. I often sense a shift within hours and always within a day. Sometimes I simply lose the insecurity or the pique passes quite naturally. Other times, past interactions come to mind and I "hear" my own comments in a different way, one that enables me to understand my friend's position.

Of course distant treatment is not a magic wand that reglues broken bonds; sometimes balance requires letting go. Reiki can help you recognize what is timely and support your healing as you move on.

Self-Inquiry

Self-inquiry is a powerful spiritual practice that helps us witness our behavior and examine our motivations without slipping into pseudo-psychology. As daily Reiki practice increases your self-awareness, you may notice places where you are unusually intolerant or you have an unwarranted amount of emotion (family members often help us find these places, and then say we're defensive!). Or maybe you are contemplating a course of action but feel unclear about the ethics. Try sending a distant treatment to the situation. Occasionally I have insights during the treatment, but more often the breakthroughs come at odd moments of my day, when my mind is busy elsewhere and too distracted to head off the self-discovery. The treatment seems to unblock an inner radiance, and I can count on feeling a shift within twenty-four hours. Reiki-supported self-inquiry can be a powerful support in times of crisis, helping us stay inwardly aligned and creating a source of trust and patience as challenging situations unfold. Whereas self-analysis can be a mental exercise that actually keeps us removed from our emotions, Reiki-supported self-inquiry anchors us in our deepest well-being and allows the self-judgment or congested past emotion to gently unravel from within. Self-inquiry is the fine art of taking stock without judging that allows us to continually open into deeper self-awareness and acceptance.

Blessing Endeavors

Whether we are creating new buildings or new organizations, using Second Degree treatment as each new entity comes into existence can help prevent problems down the line by supporting balance at each stage of the process. Even as we formulate initial plans, we can connect with Reiki to enhance alignment and clarify our direction. In this way, we can help our new creation be in harmony with its environment.

Healing Lists

With two hands, we can offer First Degree Reiki to a maximum of two people at once, with one hand on each person. Second Degree enables us to multiply our hands to offer Reiki simultaneously to more than two people. How many more? That's really up to you. You can keep a healing list where you write the names of people who have asked you for healing and send a distant treatment to the "list." The sky is the limit, but I suggest you limit yourself to a number that feels meaningful to you. If you use healing lists to extend your reach beyond the threshold of your experience of Reiki, you will likely lose confidence. Keep it simple.

REGARDING ETHICS AND PROSCRIPTIONS FOR DISTANT HEALING

Hands-on practice has some inherent boundaries: we can offer Reiki only to people we have permission to touch. As Second Degree students move into the possibility of offering Reiki without touch, Reiki goes undercover. There are no boundaries. We can offer Reiki to anyone we want, anytime we want. We may mistakenly feel we have an obligation to do so. But it's not really a matter of what you can or can't do, it's a matter of common sense and staying present.

Concerns about what we can or should do become clearer the more deeply we understand healing. I offer my students, and I offer you, contemplations that I myself use repeatedly to stay engaged in an ever-deepening inquiry into healing and Reiki.

- What is healing?
- Who is the healer?
- What is it that is healed?

In the last session of my Second Degree class, we contemplate these three questions. We sit quietly and in-drawn, notebooks and pens set aside but within reach. For those who do not have experience with contemplation, I offer these instructions:

Prepare by sitting quietly for a few moments. Give your mind a chance to settle.

Simply hold the question in your awareness, allowing your inner wisdom to percolate up through it. Let your mind be soft and open to inspiration, which may arrive in the form of words or a visual or even a memory or sound. Don't judge what occurs to you; stay open, attentive, and steady. It may be helpful to visualize or otherwise imagine this process happening in your heart.

Contemplation is not analysis. We ask and wait, not for answers but for an inner response, which may be elusive or nonverbal. Even if there are words, if you have accessed your wisdom, there is a profound experience connected to the words, a sense of the truth to which words can only point. The same words may reappear at different times accompanied by new insights.

These are questions that I return to repeatedly. Each time I contemplate these questions, I have an experience that expands my understanding. There are no "correct" answers to these questions. Continual contemplation will unearth insight into the vast healing process, and keep us fresh in our approach. The moment we stop asking ourselves "What is healing?" we become mere technicians.

My goal as a Reiki master is to support my students in creating such an intimate relationship with Reiki that ultimately there are no doubts about when to use it. The contemplations on healing help deepen our relationship with Reiki and remove doubt. So does regular practice.

But if someone feels unsure, he is less likely to practice. For students who are more comfortable with rules, I offer a guideline with which to start practice: Send Reiki only to people who have specifically asked for it, or from whom you have received permission.

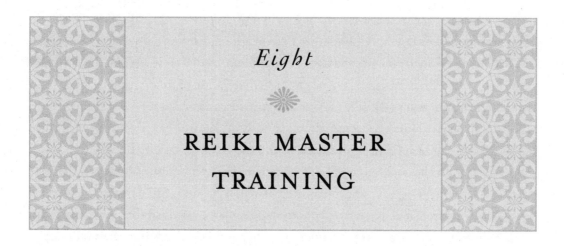

Eight

REIKI MASTER
TRAINING

Only he who obeys can command.

RIG VEDA

A Second Degree practitioner trained by another Reiki master once said to me, "Your fees are so much higher than mine. Why would anyone come to you instead of me?" Without stopping to breathe, she continued to formulate her own answer. "I guess since you're a Reiki master, you do more than I do."

"Actually," I replied, "I do less."

And so it is. A Reiki master isn't someone who has mastered Reiki, but rather someone who keeps offering herself deeply to her practice; someone who is content to do what is hers to do and leave the rest to Reiki. As a friend of mine once observed, "You're not such a great healer, you just know how to follow directions!"

Following directions is a big part of it; knowing when to ask is another. So is the discipline of continually monitoring my state and my awareness of Reiki. This helps me stay connected to the inner source of Reiki in the center of the heart. There is still much for me to learn in this area, but as I have practiced over two decades, it's become obvious that the less I do and the quieter I am inside, the more room there is for Reiki. I check inside my heart to notice what Reiki is doing, and then align myself with that. How to do this? That process is not so easily shared. Years of meditation practice have helped, and I expect it's a skill I'll refine as long as I'm alive.

Through practice and contemplation, each Reiki master can live from that pure open space in the heart that is authentic and which cannot be faked. Ideally, a Reiki master lives with the conviction of her practice, relying on practice to deepen the connection to that heart space, and to reconnect when needed. She is strong and clear without being positional. Respectful of others, she takes responsibility for her actions, never using Reiki as an excuse for a decision she's made or an action she's taken. She is comfortable sitting in silence and listening.

As Reiki masters, we all come to form our own unique relationship with Reiki, living with the reality that healing happens in a profound way when we touch, that our touch carries an authenticity we cannot control, that people's lives change when we touch them, especially when we touch for initiation. I can always tell accomplished masters because they speak of Reiki's simplicity. There is less to do and less agitation. A seasoned master is patient, confident, and has the courage to do only what is needed and leave the healing to Reiki.

TAKATA: A MODEL OF MASTERY

A Reiki master today would do well to take Hawayo Takata as her model. Takata imbibed Reiki. She carried this spiritual healing practice out of its culture of origin, transplanted it in foreign soil, and inspired her students to carry it forth to the world. Her student the Canadian Reiki master Barbara Brown said, "Takata never broke her own rules."[1] Those who knew Takata still speak of her with profound respect and admiration.

Paul David Mitchell, another one of Takata's master students, remembers arriving at his First Degree class feeling that everyone but him could do this. The only experience he had during the initiation was his arms getting really tired as he held them in the air. However, Mitchell said, "I felt carried by what she imparted through her embodiment of Reiki." He understood that it was his responsibility to practice, and that if he practiced in a disciplined way, giving himself daily treatment, he would grow in Reiki.

After his initiation as a master, Mitchell found himself in a paradoxical place where he had lots of doubts about his own abilities but no doubts about what he had received from Takata. He knew he had everything he needed, but he also knew there was much he didn't know. Mitchell told me, "I had the tools that I needed to impart this practice to others, to initiate, teach hand positions, how to treat myself and others, some commonsense things, and the principles—that's all I needed and all they needed."

It's a rare Reiki master who carries Reiki as Takata did. Not everyone was drawn to her personality, but that was never the point. Maybe no one today can match her clarity and confidence, but as a woman who lived so recently, Takata can be a model to point the direction toward mastery within each of us. The greatest value we can gain from knowing details of Takata's teaching is not to ape her personality or manner, but to be inspired by her long and unwavering devotion to practice. That was the source of her strength and authenticity. If we follow her example of daily practice, we will also, each in our own way, become strong clear models of Reiki.

WHY BECOME A REIKI MASTER?

Traditionally, being a Reiki master is very much a lifestyle, one for which there is no guidebook. Mastery itself is fluid and ever-developing. Each of us expresses our mastery according to our personalities, our circumstances, and especially, our understanding of Reiki. It is not necessary, for example, to be a vegetarian. Takata was not. She even ate red meat, albeit sparingly. Takata loved to play golf. I prefer walking and yoga. Someone else may play tennis. It doesn't matter.

What does matter is that we create a lifestyle committed to balance. It's a lot like juggling, with the balls turning into clubs, saucers, or even fire sticks without warning—

a game without rules, one in which awareness and intuition are mainstays. Reiki mastery involves a commitment to spirit, to developing one's unique spirituality.

Is there a formula for mastery? I think not. But there are some elements worth contemplating whether you are choosing a master to train you as a master, assessing the potential of a master candidate, or evaluating your own mastery.

Our primary obligation as Reiki masters is, first, to impart the love of this practice and, second, to teach the practice as we have learned it. When a student takes me as his teacher, it means he is asking me to lay the foundation for practice and guide his continuing inquiry into Reiki.

As Reiki masters, we can model masterful studentship, taking full responsibility for our choices and actions even as we open more and more profoundly to the inner radiant state we call Reiki.

As Reiki masters, what we *don't* say is at least as important as what we *do* say. We can offer a welcoming, clear introduction to Reiki practice and then humbly allow Reiki to take it from there.

Being a Reiki master does not mean being isolated, invulnerable, and closed to support. It means taking full responsibility for one's life, living in a balance of independence and interdependence, honoring the contributions that others make to us, seeking them in a timely manner, and accepting them graciously. Regular self-treatment, receiving healing from others, and having a spiritual practice provide invaluable support in the life of any student of Reiki and become even more important at the level of mastery.

HOW DOES ONE TRAIN TO BECOME A REIKI MASTER?

Once you decide to become a Reiki master, you need to find a master who meets your requirements and who will accept you as a master candidate. If this is the master who has already trained you in First and Second Degree, you are fortunate. If not, you have some work ahead of you.

First decide what kind of training you want. Traditional Reiki master training involves mutual recognition between the initiating master and the candidate, a period of time in which they get to know each other if they don't already. Reiki master and candidate agree to respect each other and to value their relationship. The details of how this plays out will be different for each duo and may change enormously as the candidate matures in her mastery.

Usually, the student is first trained in the skills of mastery. Then comes the actual initiation, followed by some level of supervision. Traditional masters tend to consider only candidates who are already functioning as Reiki professionals, offering considerable treatment in a variety of situations (in their private work space, in hospitals, or through home visits) and who are comfortable speaking publicly about Reiki. Being a Reiki master is a profession as well as a calling. Masters need to have enough business experience to organize and promote classes and keep track of fees and expenses.

Finally, it's best that mastery develop on a foundation of living masterfully. If we're not yet managing the basic details of our own lives well, how can we take on the added responsibility of initiating and mentoring others? Give yourself the time you need to prepare yourself for this powerful life transition.

If training in the traditional way, master candidates can expect to sit in on a number of classes taught by the initiating master and to organize classes for their master to teach. Some initiating masters co-teach with a new master, but supervision can also be arranged in other ways. Master candidates need to learn certain information, such as how to structure classes and how to perform initiations.

Reiki master candidates need to develop a lifestyle that supports an ever-deepening relationship with Reiki, if they don't already have one. Important decisions may arise, and the continued mentoring of the initiating master can be invaluable.

Some masters are very structured and demand that their candidates conform to their methodology. Others are more improvisational. One approach is not inherently better than another, but the match between a master's teaching style and a candidate's temperament and learning style is best considered as part of the original decision to work together.

Part apprentice, part protégé, the candidate has a unique arrangement with the Reiki master. I'm not in favor of formalizing the process into a curriculum as if it were an academic training. Some people need more training and some less. Some masters become working partners with masters they have trained, at least for a time.

In accepting a master candidate, I look for someone who shares my values and has the commitment and the tools to self-monitor and self-reference. I prefer the candidate to have an ongoing daily spiritual practice in addition to Reiki. I'm not looking to rubber-stamp masters or create clones. I'm looking for someone strong in himself, who makes decisions carefully, who looks honestly within to discern truth from opinion, who is comfortable with silence and space and uncertainty, who relies on practice and looks to the precepts for direction.

CHOOSING A REIKI MASTER TO TRAIN YOU AS A MASTER

Now that there are so many options, it is particularly important for master candidates to carefully choose the master and the conditions under which they will be initiated and trained. Particularly consider whether the initiating master trains in a way that is consonant with her professed values. Contemplate whether your master is offering you the support that you need to begin your practice. Some prominent Reiki masters are in demand like a brand name, but I encourage master candidates to look beyond the prestige and choose a master who can deliver what the individual candidate needs both to learn the material attached to mastery and to continue developing in Reiki. There may be a Reiki master less well known but closer to home and more available who is a good choice for you.

A satisfying training will likely be an intimate experience. When choosing your Reiki master or deciding to accept the invitation he offers to train you, contemplate the potential for relationship. What kinds of relationships do you see this master having? How does he carry himself in the world? How does he treat people—everyone, not just his candidates?

Look for a Reiki master who has accomplished considerable healing in her own being. How can we tell? We all feel it when someone is comfortable in her skin, accepting of others, clear without being judgmental. Perhaps most important, look for a master who has healthy boundaries, one who, rather than trying to create you in his own image, will support you to become the Reiki master that only you can be, offering you guidance at points of challenge and, above all, referring you back to your relationship with Reiki again and again.

We don't attain mastery when we receive the master initiation; we merely begin our path toward mastery. We've passed the entrance exam, but we are just starting the course work, a lot of which may occur in the school of hard knocks.

Even if the relationship doesn't unfold as you had hoped, as was the case for me, engaging in relationship with your Reiki master is a valuable part of your training. If you reach a point where it is healthy to move on, do so. But above all, practice, practice, practice. If you persist in your practice, if you let Reiki show you how to live from your depths, there will be a point at which your outer teacher will give way to the inner teacher. If your Reiki master is both skilled and seasoned, she will have this transition in mind from the beginning. She will anticipate it and support it. The Reiki master is both a teacher in that she gives you the technique (the master symbol, the knowledge of the initiations, practical knowledge) and a guide for the unfolding of the process that begins with initiation. That's why it's called initiation. It starts something.

Your Reiki master can't make you a Reiki master. He can only give you the initiation. You have to do the work, which may involve dismantling the scaffolding of judgments that have offered you protection and support as you grew over many years. True mastery, one based on daily self-practice, offers the opportunity to move beyond these temporary and rather arbitrary supports, to live from one's center. There is a transition as you dissolve the old supports that may take a long time. It doesn't happen all at once; but with continuing practice over time, just as surely as dripping water dissolves rock, Reiki will deepen your understanding and soften your heart toward yourself and others.

OTHER FORMATS FOR TRAINING

As with First and Second Degree, Reiki master training is available in a dizzying range of formats. No matter how great or insignificant you think Reiki is, there is a training that will reflect the value you place on Reiki. There are formats that offer Reiki master training in a week, a weekend, an afternoon, or online. More surprising than the fact that there are opportunities to become instant Reiki masters is the fact that people sign up for these opportunities. Before you sign up, please consider this: How can mastery of anything be developed in a week, in a weekend, or in an afternoon?

No great path speaks of fast fast fast. In his PBS presentation *Healing and the Mind,* Bill Moyers interviewed a t'ai chi master in Beijing who required aspiring students to show up for training at dawn every morning for three years before he would accept them as students. Another renowned master practiced for ten years before he felt *chi.*

Can initiation be done in absentia? Yes. Is this the best way for it to happen? In most cases, probably not. In the best scenario, the Reiki master serves not only as the catalyst of initiation but also as the one who provides technical training and who mentors the student. When initiation happens in absentia, such as over the Internet, these valuable functions are lost.

FEES

Takata clearly envisioned being a Reiki master as a career and chose $10,000 as the fee for master initiation and training. Remember, Takata was prepared to sell her house to pay for her Reiki training. After Takata's death in 1980, the twenty-two Reiki masters she trained continued to use her fee structure. Within a decade after her death, however, some Reiki masters no longer honored Takata's standards for both training and fee. As with First and Second Degree, an array of Reiki master training options is currently available at a wide range of fees.

I could never have imagined as a new Reiki master where this practice would take me. Although $10,000 was then the most money I had ever spent in one place at one time, I have never felt that I overpaid for my training. Nor do I know a practicing Reiki master who paid $10,000 for traditional training and felt he paid too much. I have heard a lot of defensiveness from masters who have paid less—even masters with well-established, thoughtful practices—as if the choice to pay $10,000 of our own money is somehow inherently wrong. I find it curious, the drama about money. After all, we cannot buy mastery. We pay for the initiation and training; mastery is earned only through practice.

Bethal Phaigh, a Reiki master trained by Takata, wrote of meeting a respected kahuna, a traditional Hawaiian healer elder, in her unpublished manuscript, "Journey into Consciousness." They spoke of training healers. I was struck by how closely his remarks mirrored the progression of Reiki training. He said most people could learn the basic level, in which one learned how to relate to nature. In the next stage, the student learned the healing secrets of the plants. But the kahuna would not attempt to share the advanced teachings with many. He said, "I will not try to teach others what it has taken me forty years to learn unless they are ready to dedicate their lives to it."

FOR REIKI MASTERS WHO ARE READY TO TRAIN REIKI MASTERS

Once you become a Reiki master, your life will change in both subtle and obvious ways. Give yourself time to get used to your new relationship with Reiki. When you start teaching, devote yourself to First and Second Degree classes for a while. These are the levels of practice that you have been practicing, so you have a lot of personal experience to draw from. Why accept a Reiki master student before you have at least as much experience being a Reiki master as you do practicing Second Degree?

Just as I wasn't drawn to less expensive Reiki master trainings, I'm not comfortable charging less than I paid. However, a student's willingness to pay my fee is not enough to qualify her as a master candidate. I have been approached by students wanting to pay me $10,000 to initiate them and quickly teach them the mechanics of initiating others. As of this writing, I have yet to agree to that, perhaps because none of these students showed the depth of reliance on practice that is the cornerstone of mastery. As the student committed to daily practice moves toward mastery, the commitment to practice paves the way to reliance on one's practice.

Training students at any level is not about the money. I only want to train master students who truly value both Reiki and what I have to offer as a Reiki master. I look for students who have a relationship with Reiki that is grounded in practice and self-responsibility. I want to know that I will be proud of my students' future decisions, even if I don't agree with them, because they are so deeply engaged with Reiki. If I feel that a student has the potential for mastery but is not ready, I'll share that assessment. If asked, I'll offer guidance as to how he might develop his readiness, but it's up to the student to prepare himself for mastery, not me. It's only my job to initiate and train him once we both agree on the timing.

Training at every level is customized to the students present. In the First and Second Degree classes, that customization takes place within the structure of the class. Takata didn't leave a structure for training masters, and her masters didn't have elaborate training. They usually organized classes for her, sat in on other classes, and had some continuing access to her mentoring. More than anything, the twenty-two masters Takata trained had her unwavering example of living Reiki mastery and continuing Reiki practice.

If you commit to training a master, remember that we are Reiki masters, not taskmasters. Reiki master Helen Haberly, who studied First and Second Degree with Takata, described her as having "a ready smile with a quiet humor, finding much to amuse her in life. Because she was very alert and quick-witted, little escaped her attention. An excellent judge of people, her assessments were at times uncomfortably accurate, although she seldom voiced any personal criticism. Instead, she focused on the positive and offered compliments whenever possible."[2]

If something needs to be said, say it with detachment and kindness. Everyone wants to grow. It's enough to gently identify the need or point the way. If the Reiki master tries to control every step, no one will grow—not the master candidate and not the master. If we feel burdened, it's time for self-inquiry regarding boundaries and how we are carrying our mastery.

A master's decision to train a Reiki master will depend on his definition of the master/student relationship. Those who feel it changes the power dynamics between two people may be wise to avoid mixing this relationship with personal relationships. If as a master, you have any doubts about accepting a particular candidate, just check up inside. Don't assume that everything that looks like resistance is something to be overcome. It may be best not to enter into an agreement to train a master unless you feel a clear inner go-ahead. Seasoned masters become more comfortable in trusting their intuition. If there is an inner stop sign, don't personalize it or project it onto the candidate. It may just not be timely or not a good match, for reasons that may remain unknown. If you don't trust the candidate's process, don't take his money.

If master and candidate each take responsibility for their own wellness and integrity, training a master can be a rewarding experience for both. Think of the yearlong apprenticeship as a guideline only. Give each student what he needs, which may be more or less than what either the student or the master has in mind. Framing the relationship between Reiki master and candidate with unnecessary formality may create unnecessary problems. When there are difficulties, it's often because we're seeing the situation in flat either/or dimensions. Moving to the fuller perspective of "both," something that Reiki helps us accomplish, helps restore balance and flow to the relationship.

Master training can bring up authority issues for both student and master. If this is happening, perhaps the master isn't yet ready to be training masters. If a master is aligned with Reiki, she carries Reiki's authority comfortably and doesn't precipitate power struggles. A Reiki master is not a guru. Reiki is the real teacher; the master is a mentor.

Like the parent of an adult child, the initiating Reiki master is wise to step back and let the masters he's initiated seek his mentoring as they feel the need. Their mastery is between them and Reiki, and the initiating master needn't hover.

THE VALUE OF TIME

An inner knowing that is not academic develops with mastery over time. We simply become more comfortable with mystery. As we let go of the need to know and understand that this need keeps us from being deeply present—because part of us is always ruminating and thinking—a different kind of knowing emerges and evolves. As we become content with listening, we gain confidence that we know what we need to know when we need to know it, and we are confirmed in mastery. This process takes time and cannot be circumvented. Mastery is a solitary position. We are alone in mystery and we are that.

Nine

REIKI PRACTICE:
CREATING
CONTINUING
SUPPORT

Give a man a fish and you feed him for a day.
Teach him to fish and you feed him for a lifetime.

LAO TZU

When I began learning Reiki during my first months of pregnancy, I was feeling the usual first-trimester blahs, and was tired and nauseated every waking hour. Perhaps because I stumbled upon Reiki when I was feeling so low, my enthusiasm for practice was strong from Day One. For me, learning Reiki was like the beginning of a romance. I fit Reiki into stolen moments throughout my day and could hardly wait to give myself a full treatment. A couple of friends practiced on me occasionally, especially once my daughter was born, but most of the Reiki I received came from my own hands. It was sweet and refreshing and profound. The pleasure of self-treatment and the obvious benefits it brought fueled my practice. I didn't have to discipline myself to practice because I relished my Reiki time.

THE GIFTS DAILY PRACTICE BRINGS

Reiki clears the mind, restores the body, and refreshes the spirit. You don't have to take my word for it. You can try it yourself. It doesn't take long to notice. After all, the mind is not a self-cleaning oven that automatically burns the spillover from our life's experiences to ash. The residue of negative experiences and unresolved emotions lingers, often affecting us in ways we don't recognize. We never leave the house without combing our hair or brushing our teeth. Reiki gives us a way to brush the debris from our mind and spirit as well.

When we're young, we feel that time is our friend. We don't realize, as my meditation teacher once said, that we are not spending time—time is spending us. Our bodies are resilient, and we get away with a lot. We don't have to make much daily effort to feel good, and so we usually don't. As we get older, though, the resilience in our bodies diminishes. If we don't create healing on a daily basis, we quickly feel the difference. And the aging process doesn't just affect us physically. We lose mental clarity and can't remember where we left our memory. Emotionally we become brittle and fearful. If we're smart, we begin to appreciate that every little thing we do to support our well-being matters.

What if we had that understanding *before* our bodies aged? Do you think we would be more motivated to practice daily? How profound are the benefits of daily practice that we cannot see? Though they may seem inconsequential, the invisible benefits of Reiki are in many ways the most consequential because they are preventive. It has always been curious to me when people who are already suffering experience the benefits of Reiki and then stop their daily practice once they're feeling better. You don't need a psychic to predict the future in that scenario. Chris Conairis, an Anusara yoga teacher in Tucson, Arizona, encourages his students with these wise words: "Practice now, when you don't need to, so that when you are in need, you won't come up short."

If you're good at light housekeeping, you intuitively understand the benefits of daily practice. If, on the other hand, you wait until the floors are scummy so you can have fun scraping them, daily practice is going to be a challenge, but a challenge worth meeting. Let's stay with the housekeeping example. If you can equate the impact of soot on your windowsills being blown into your home every time you open the windows with the accumulation of stress in your system, you're well on your way to being motivated to give yourself Reiki treatment every day of your life.

There are so many reasons why daily practice makes a difference. Anyone who has received regular care, whether seeing a therapist or getting a weekly massage or even a pedicure, knows how much it means knowing you have that special time in your schedule. If you give yourself Reiki at a certain time of your day, every day, you relax into that rhythm of care. With daily practice, you know you'll never go longer than twenty-four hours without returning to center.

One of the most valuable benefits that comes from daily practice is dissolving the roots of negative behaviors and emotions. This takes time. Since I started practicing Reiki, I have found myself in situations in which I had been afraid in the past. Although I no longer felt fearful, I could still feel the skeleton of the habit of fear vibrating inside me on the brink of manifesting. But I also felt confident that the transformation would continue as long as I continued my daily practice.

Life is challenging at times even for students who practice daily self-treatment. But if we have a steady practice, we feel secure that we have the wherewithal to sustain ourselves. When we practice self-treatment regularly, the difficulties don't overwhelm our lives; they just feel like details. If we are not practicing, life's difficulties more easily become burdensome; they take over our perspective, and we become ineffectual. Daily practice enables us to embody our highest values.

CONTINUING SELF-TREATMENT

Reiki is as natural as a mother's touch, and I love that it's so normal and uncomplicated. But as normal and simple as Reiki is, it requires the effort of daily practice to optimize its benefits. Consciously developing a habit of daily practice will extract Reiki's natural goodness and nourish you every day.

I ask my First Degree students to commit to six months of daily practice. My hope is that within that amount of time, they will become so enamored of their practice that they will continue. After six months, a student can look back and clearly see the differences that Reiki has made in his life. Because that's why we practice, for the cumulative benefit, not simply the pleasure of an individual treatment.

Most of my yoga practice sessions are not about building strength or mastering a new posture; they are simply about practicing yoga today. I may feel wonderful after any particular yoga session, and that's a good thing, but it does not represent the benefit I receive from practicing yoga regularly. It's the same with Reiki. Some days bring amazing Reiki experiences. Most days I simply practice.

So I sweetly but clearly state my request for a six-month commitment to daily practice early in the class. It's important that students understand from the beginning that, without practice, the benefits they experience from the class fade into memory, gobbled up by the jaws of daily stress.

The following are a few questions that predictably emerge in my classes regarding daily practice:

- *"Do I really have to practice every day?"*

    I see this question on the face of First Degree students, some of whom have never committed to doing anything other than eating every day! Well, Reiki is like eating. It nourishes us even more profoundly than food. It relaxes us more deeply than sleep. It replenishes the spirit. It's not that you *have* to do it every day; it's that you *get* to. The answer to this question is an unequivocal "Yes." We practice every day. That's why it's called practice.

- *"But I've never been very disciplined. How can I possibly hope to maintain a daily practice?"*

    I admire the sincerity of students who ask this question. They are probably the ones who least have to worry about keeping their commitment. The answer is easy. Any day that you aren't able to do your regular practice, just make it a point to fall asleep with one or both hands on your body. Of course we don't want that to be all that we do regularly (although that's better than not practicing at all), but sometimes life gets ahead of us and falling asleep with Reiki maintains our practice. And if you stop practicing, remember that you can simply begin again at any time.

- *"Will I lose Reiki if I don't practice?"*

   No, you won't. If you have four initiations in First Degree practice (check with your Reiki master), you cannot lose Reiki. The worst you can do is to fail to develop your Reiki by not practicing regularly. But even so, when tough times come, as they do in life, Reiki will be there for you. Takata taught that the secret of capability is how much you practice.[1] If you do not practice, you will not have the same capacity for Reiki that you would if you had practiced regularly. Nor will you have the same resilience in your system as if you had been taking care of yourself all along. You will also not have the confidence in Reiki that daily practice creates. But you will still be able to access Reiki through your hands.

Practice Reiki the way you put on your seat belt in the car. You don't think about whether or not you feel like it; you just do it. Let Reiki be your seat belt for life, keeping you close to center.

Since Reiki is so open and flexible, it's helpful if we are self-aware and disciplined. Create your daily treatment as a haven by choosing a time of day when you can always at least place hands for a few minutes.

WHEN PRACTICE BECOMES ROUTINE

When we first practice Reiki, there are usually a lot of new sensations. Sometimes the sensations can be quite strong, and it's easy to assume that means Reiki is activated more strongly. The fact is, we don't know that. It's important to separate the *sensations* of Reiki from the actual *workings* of Reiki. What we feel is superficial compared to everything that happens during Reiki treatment. After a while, the sensations felt during daily practice become less dramatic because there is not so much realignment needed. But when the experience of Reiki is quiet, it may be that the most profound healing is being accomplished. As we practice watching patiently, the discipline of relaxed attention and the effects of Reiki together will expand our awareness. Remember, we practice not for entertainment but for the accumulated benefit. As in any long-term relationship, there will be times when you take Reiki for granted or find it boring. But there will also be times of rediscovery and deepened intimacy.

Because we are creatures of habit, it helps to have a form to our practice. We honor the teachers who initiated us into the practice by adopting their form. Practicing as we have been taught protects our investment and allows it to mature with interest. After all, if we change the practice, how can we be sure we are receiving the full benefit? Only practice reveals the depth of this healing art and develops its mature power.

Reiki master Helen Haberly wrote *Reiki: Hawayo Takata's Story.* According to Haberly, sometimes Takata said to start treatment with the head, other times the abdomen, or she might say it didn't matter where you started as long as you gave the full treatment.

Let your hands develop a Reiki habit. If you follow a sequence through all the placements, your hands know where to go next and treatment requires no more thought than to remember to start. If you can't practice as you were taught because of physical limitations such as restricted mobility or chronic pain, modify the sequence to meet your needs and let that be your sequence.

As we continue to practice daily, there are times when we feel as if nothing is happening. We can certainly shorten our practice time, but we shortchange ourselves if we completely stop. Just because we don't feel anything doesn't mean nothing is happening. It's likely that the sessions when we don't notice anything are actually when the most important work, the work of prevention, is being done! During those quiet times Reiki may be balancing our biofield. Maintaining ourselves at this level is like wiping the furniture long before we can draw our name in the dust. So when you have a "quiet" practice session, rather than assuming nothing worthwhile is happening, realize that's when persevering in your daily practice will earn the best return on your investment. This subtle level is always happening, but when there are greater levels of imbalance, the rebalancing can be very dramatic. We notice that and think, *Wow, wow, wow!* We of course get excited by what we can notice, but let reason remind us that more is happening. And as we persevere in our practice, our awareness will expand and we will notice more.

Intention—staying mindful of our goal—and the conviction built from our past experience with Reiki carry us through and minimize the backsliding that happens in the best of practices. They enable us to accept our practice even when it is uneventful, to persevere and simply begin again.

Sometimes I hear Reiki students say there came a time when they needed something stronger than Reiki. I have never felt this, and it puzzled me for a long time. Then I realized that I had persisted in my practice despite the highs and lows of sensation. I was in it for the long haul and didn't give up when Reiki didn't give me the experience I thought I should be having. I practiced even when I didn't feel like practicing. I wasn't rigid about it; my practice has always been quite fluid. There are times when I've done two hours of Reiki a day and times when I've done considerably less. But I have given myself treatment on a daily basis, with the understanding that the practice is larger than what I know, and that my relationship with Reiki was growing even when I couldn't see it. If Reiki is your first experience of practice, you may need a little discipline and patience. If you never practice regularly, you'll never know how beneficial it is and how gratifying it can be. There are always days when we practice not because we feel like it but just because we said we would.

When your enthusiasm is lagging, make it fun. Give yourself a treatment while watching a movie or listening to your favorite music, or get together with a Reiki friend. The structure and delightful sound of my Reiki chime timer is enough to engage me on those mornings when I'm just not in the mood. (See www.ReikiInMedicine.org under Resources.) Don't cheat yourself. Keep practicing.

YOUR DEVELOPING INTUITION

Intuition develops naturally as we continually connect with consciousness through daily practice. Many students notice it even during the First Degree class. It's probably not so much a matter of having more intuition as that there is less "static" in our minds. Reiki practice makes us quieter inside, and we notice our inner reality more often. The more connected and centered we feel, the more likely we are to hear the intuition that has always been there.

Takata encouraged her students to be intuitive in their practice, while being mindful of the practice form. You can let your hands linger where they feel active, or use a placement other than you were taught if your hands feel drawn to do so. As long as your touch is appropriate, you can follow your hands. Takata said, "Reiki will guide you. Let the Reiki hands find it. They will know what to do."[2] The Japanese word for this intuitive practice is *reiji*. You will know when/if this happens (and nothing is lost by simply practicing the basic treatment). Although everyone has his own experience, you become aware that your hands have a direct relationship with Reiki that doesn't go through your mind, as if your hands have become Reiki.

Claire came to Second Degree class concerned about the psychic experiences her friends were having as they practiced Reiki. The mere thought of it made her uncomfortable, but she also wondered why it wasn't happening to her. Claire didn't know if she was more afraid of having the experiences or worried about not having them. If you can relate to this, just remember that everyone has her own relationship with Reiki, and that Takata did not teach psychic exercises in Second Degree training.

When offering Reiki to ourselves or to another, we may get to eavesdrop on the inner conversation. Sometimes we hear more and sometimes it may be muffled. Think carefully before you share your experience or observations with the friend you've just treated. For one thing, it takes years to be sure you're accessing pure intuition (a steady meditation practice helps). Second, the person may feel violated, too vulnerable and exposed. She came for a treatment, not a reading. Trust that Reiki alone will do what is needed, and keep your experiences to yourself.

A Second Degree student of mine was looking for people to practice on. The mother of my son's friend was interested in Reiki, so I connected the two of them. The mother called me later to thank me . . . and to vent. Despite the many warnings

I had given about sharing "insights" after giving treatment, my student had made a comment that left the woman feeling violated. It took a lot of listening to defuse the lingering upset. Some practitioners would pass it off as part of the healing, but frankly, I find that attitude irresponsible. Yes, not everyone gets along easily, and some people naturally grate on one another's nerves. But if the practitioner limits her conversation to meet-and-greet, there's no hook on which the Reiki recipient can hang this irritation (which may not stop him from trying).

Pay attention. Pay attention inside and pay attention outside. Learn the difference between intuition and imagination, and especially between intuition and projection. Learn to discern the vibration of truth and the vibration of fantasy. Give it time.

REIKI AS SPIRITUAL PRACTICE

Reiki is a spiritual healing practice in that it accesses consciousness. However, whether Reiki is a spiritual practice or not depends on what we bring to our practice. Do you practice regularly with commitment and gratitude? Do you observe your practice and yourself and contemplate your experiences?

Spiritual practice does not require belief, nor does it mean that we renounce critical thinking. On the contrary, as we open ourselves to increasingly expanded, subtle states, it is important to contemplate our experiences and use our intellect to refine our understanding, to uncover the true essence, release the distortions, and review our lives in the context of what we have experienced to be true. We open to inner experiences and then use our critical thinking to understand how to apply those realizations to our lives. It's like breathing. We take the air in, our bodies take what we can use, and we exhale what's left. We don't just keep inhaling inhaling inhaling until we explode! We open our subtle awareness, knowing that distortion can seep in with an experience. We apply critical thinking, even as we are aware of the limits of logic.

As our relationship with Reiki develops with committed practice over time, the distinction between Reiki pulsations and Reiki consciousness blurs. The practitioner becomes aware of being anchored in that ineffable state, or even catching glimpses of it, at times when Reiki is not being practiced. Physicians and other professional care-givers find this tremendously supportive, lifting them out of the sea of demands that clinical care-giving can become. They feel supported by a silent partner that encompasses the relationship with the patient rather than pitting them against one another.

Those of us who are not health-care professionals experience this spiritual support in ways that are meaningful in our own lives. A Reiki student in the Middle East e-mailed me with a question. The note was written in limited English; his message was uplifting: "I learn there is no need to search for truth because it comes to us as we open our hearts through this beautiful practice."

SHARING REIKI

Giving Reiki to someone else or to a pet is in many ways like giving Reiki to yourself, but different. Some of us have ample opportunities to share Reiki, but others don't. Feel free to share Reiki or not, as is comfortable. But plan ahead. Don't leave your First Degree class without connecting to someone you feel drawn to. In this way you'll have a comfortable Reiki buddy to trade treatment with when and if you want. Having the shared class experience will help you get past the "Am I doing this right?" awkwardness. I also have students practice on each other during class so that they will feel less shy outside of class.

Once your First Degree class is finished, be aware that there is no rush to treat others. Self-treatment is most important, and you'll want to start that immediately. According to Canadian Reiki master Rick Bockner, Takata encouraged her students to start with self-treatment daily and then offer Reiki to the people and animals around them and see where it goes from there. Whenever you feel drawn to share Reiki with family or friends, here are a few suggestions to help you get started.

Mindfully and Gently

Sharing Reiki with another student from your class makes the transition to practicing on others very comfortable. But if you don't have a Reiki buddy, and you feel like offering Reiki to someone else, just take the time to approach the situation mindfully. If you hear yourself thinking, "So-and-so really needs this," do everyone a favor and stop right there. Anyone can benefit from Reiki but not everyone is going to be drawn to it, especially if they feel that it's being shoved down their throats. Avoid coming at someone with the attitude that you are going to fix her—it's a great way to add tension to your relationship, and your friend may refuse your offer outright. Nor is it helpful to intimidate friends into receiving Reiki, even if they are sick—especially if they are sick. Even in families, Reiki can become a political issue if the Reiki student feels an emotional need to share it with her spouse/child/parent (fill in the blank). Remember, first give Reiki to yourself, and then quite naturally to whoever else shows up. (Takata told a story on herself of giving Reiki to a woman who was seasick and inadvertently putting her hand on the woman's billfold, causing the woman to scream for help![3])

Preparing a Physical Space to Comfortably Share Reiki

When offering someone a full treatment, take a few minutes to prepare the space. A covered massage table in a room free of distractions is ideal, but not necessary. You can use a studio couch or even a bed that doesn't have a footboard, if needed. People who were raised sitting on chairs instead of the ground will likely find giving treatment on the floor, as a shiatsu practitioner does, to be physically taxing. In shiatsu, the practitioner changes positions frequently and uses his body weight to work the points. Reiki practitioners place hands lightly and hold their position for many minutes, so it's most comfortable if you are sitting a bit lower than the person you're treating. Of course, if you find yourself in an awkward position, gently adjust your body (encourage your friend to do the same). There's no reason to hurt yourself offering Reiki. If you are at an odd angle that causes pain in your back, wrist, shoulder, or neck, it's only going to get worse, so gently adjust yourself as soon as you feel any discomfort. Your friend will be so relaxed that your movement won't disturb him.

The Treatment Experience —
Yours and Your Friend's

Occasionally during or after a treatment, the receiver spontaneously remembers a past experience. Sometimes while receiving Reiki, a person experiences emotion or tears for no apparent reason. Please be mindful. Let your friend know that this is all part of the natural path of healing, give her a tissue, and don't intrude. Takata-trained Reiki master Wanja Twan describes these tears poetically as being "like ice melting" and says simply, "We don't have to know." Whatever needs to be done, Twan says, "Reiki will do it gently."

Students have a wide range of responses to their first experiences of offering and receiving Reiki with someone else. Many notice the sense of timelessness, especially when receiving. Some feel a soft suction in the palms, or feel as if either their hands or their partner's body is somehow pulsing softly and invisibly. One doctor expressed feeling that her partner's hands were listening to her body. Occasionally a student reports feeling awkward, certain he's not doing it right because nothing could be so easy. Most students feel the continuity between offering and receiving Reiki, that we also receive Reiki when we place hands to give treatment to someone else.

Avoid interpreting another's experience. If asked, you can always deflect the question back to the recipient, encouraging him to contemplate the experience. Meaning is an individual matter, and continues to unfold over time. If, in times of emotion or in the sweet, open time after a session, you decide to say something, please run your words by the Four Gates of Speech. Before speaking, ask yourself, the following questions:

Is it true?
Is it kind?
Is it necessary?
Is it timely?

Sometimes there is an increase in sensation in an area where Reiki is activated strongly. If your friend is uncomfortable, explain that this is usually short-lived, and offer to move your hands. People are generally patient with these experiences, sensing that they are somehow part of a healing process. If, however, your friend is not comfortable, back off. There is no reason to force the issue. The healing process has been started, and you don't have to stay focused on it.

According to Rick Bockner and Wanja Twan, Takata thanked Reiki and the recipient at the end of the treatment.

As mentioned in earlier chapters, theoretically you don't even have to be conscious to offer Reiki. This is good news for parents who doze off Reiki-ing a child to sleep, or who sleep with a Reiki hand on an ill spouse. It's also good news for Reiki students who need surgery. Just ask one of your caregivers to place your hands on your belly as soon as it is feasible, even before you regain consciousness after surgery. Reiki's spontaneous, responsive activation is one of its greatest gifts.

CHAIR REIKI

Students often have more opportunities to share Reiki with friends through abbreviated chair treatments than through full lying-down sessions, and some students actually prefer the chair format. Don't underestimate what can happen in five or ten minutes of chair Reiki, and don't hesitate to offer even moments of Reiki first aid (while calling 911 if needed). Since Reiki is activated as needed, even an abbreviated treatment can be considered a full treatment. Stay mindful of the placements used in the full protocol, and do what you can in the situation you are in and with the time available. Especially if you don't know the person well, it may be wise to stay with the head and the shoulders. Remember Takata's words: "Do what you can. Some Reiki is better than none at all."

Always keep in mind that you are an ambassador for this practice. The people you address either will be interested in Reiki or will discount it, depending on the quality of your presentation and your ability to avoid assumptions and speak to people where they are. Consider your words carefully, and be aware of your demeanor. Is your presence welcoming?

PRACTICE CAUTIONS

Since Reiki is safe, most people who share Reiki with others have no repercussions and don't need to read this section. But if you experience any repercussions from giving treatment to another, read on.

Occasionally a momentary pang moves through the practitioner's body as he offers Reiki. As long as it is short-lived, you need not be concerned. Any lingering discomfort is the result of interacting on levels other than Reiki. If this is happening to you, contemplate the following questions:

- Are you allowing Reiki to do the work, or are you trying to "do" something?
- Are you attached to the outcome?
- Are you trying to impress someone?
- Are you appreciating the value of what you are offering?

This can be tricky, because Reiki is effortless and we are used to valuing effort. Are you results-oriented or practice-oriented? Performance goals may be appropriate for a physician evaluating a healing program of which Reiki is a component, but such goals should be held lightly by the Reiki student.

What can go awry when sharing Reiki with another? If you keep to the treatment protocol and comport yourself with integrity, nothing will go awry outwardly. But inwardly, other things may be happening. Observe how you feel during the session and afterward. If you ever feel drained, that's a clear sign that something other than Reiki is happening.

If you feel disappointed or in any way incomplete after giving Reiki treatment to others, examine how you are giving. Either we give treatment with no strings attached or we trade. If we're trading, we need to be clear what the arrangements are, not be coy and wait for our friend to bring it up. Not addressing these issues will harm relationships.

Look honestly at how you feel toward the person you're treating. Feeling sorry for someone does not heal him, and it endangers you. It creates an unequal relationship. Don't engender dependency. Protection is the ability to connect and disconnect, hands-on, hands-off.

If you have any negative experiences when giving someone else Reiki, back up. Practice more on yourself. It's possible that it's simply your relationship with a particular person that is the problem, in which case you can just refer the person elsewhere for treatment. However, if this is happening frequently, it may be your relationship with yourself that needs healing. Stop treating others and attend to your own needs through consistent Reiki self-treatment, through self-inquiry (which may involve a process of remorse and forgiveness), and through receiving healing from compassionate, experienced, nonjudgmental healers, whether they are Reiki practitioners, psychotherapists, spiritual counselors, or whatever appeals to you at the time.

KEEPING CLEAR UNDERSTANDING

Confusion can arise when a practitioner is casual with language. Then we hear statements such as "I did this" or "I did that" and words like "moving," "breaking up," "generating," or "beaming," which sound as though the Reiki practitioner is directing the healing. However, when I question practitioners who speak this way (and I always question because I want to understand), invariably they express the feeling that they are aligned with Reiki rather than making it happen. It can become even more challenging to stay with language that reflects the passivity of the Reiki practitioner as our experience of Reiki grows and flourishes, and we move into a more profound identification with Reiki consciousness. These expanded states require vigilance and discipline. No matter how expanded our subtle experience may be, we remain accountable for our actions, behavior, and demeanor. It's important to stay grounded, for everyone's sake.

Practitioners who have been educated in various models of subtle anatomy such as chakras or meridians are wise to remember not only that this is a different system but also that primordial consciousness is not confined to such constructs. Yoga master Kausthub Desikachar cautions his students to remember that primordial consciousness "has no form, no gender, no qualities, no features" and not to take constructs that are meant as educational models too literally.[4]

CONTINUING EDUCATION AND REIKI COMMUNITY

Although practice is our primary connection to Reiki, students often seek additional ways to enhance their understanding or engage in the Reiki community. I write *ReikiUpdate,* my occasional e-newsletter, to stimulate dialogue about a thoughtful approach to Reiki and to inform the community of medical research. (You can sign up at www.ReikiInMedicine.org.) You might also consider retaking a Reiki class. The basic material is the same, yet each class is unique, and your prior experience yields new insight.

I offer periodic Reiki reunions where students come to reconnect or expand their connection to Reiki. Karen, a longtime Reiki practitioner, came to one of these evenings. She had not been practicing recently. As she shared Reiki with other students, she felt deeply moved and nourished. Karen saw that she had become energetically stagnant and understood how she had hurt herself by not practicing. She also realized that she had stopped practicing Reiki because she was angry (*just for today* . . .). As she contemplated, it became clear that she was angry because she had been feeling obligated to offer Reiki to everyone around her.

It's not that Reiki turned on Karen when she stopped her practice. Rather, she had become used to experiencing the refreshment Reiki brings on a regular basis. Once she stopped practicing, she no longer had that benefit. Because Karen had practiced so long, and because she contemplated her experience, she could tell the difference. She understood what she had done, how she had created her own discomfort, how obeying her anger hurt her, and she was relieved to be practicing again.

Some communities have Reiki circles or Reiki clinics where practitioners and non-practitioners gather to share and experience Reiki. I host a monthly Reiki clinic at the Jewish Community Center on Manhattan's Upper West Side that is attended by a wide range of Reiki students and professionals, as well as by community members who are curious about Reiki. Everyone gets to lie on the table to receive a thirty-minute Reiki treatment, usually from two practitioners simultaneously. The practitioners stay for Reiki conversation and mentoring after everyone has had a treatment and the others have left. I encourage the students and practitioners to make Reiki buddies and meet on their own to share treatments. If there is either a circle or a clinic in your community, give it a try. The support of a group is always valuable, and the gratitude and feedback from people experiencing Reiki for the first time is encouraging.

If none of these options is available in your community, why not offer to help your Reiki master organize a group? Or host your own Reiki gathering, inviting other students you know. You can have an informal Reiki social like the quilting bees of pioneer times, a group of students getting together to share Reiki at whatever regular intervals suit your schedules. You don't need a Reiki master to supervise because as long as you are being considerate of one another's needs, you can't do Reiki wrong. But be mindful to simply practice together and avoid teaching.

If you ever feel disconnected from your practice for any reason, arrange to receive treatment from another practitioner, especially your Reiki master if available. You can also make a spiritual retreat either as part of your spiritual community or simply set aside time dedicated to spiritual practice, including Reiki. It can be as simple as shutting off the phone one evening and creating a simple ceremony that is meaningful to you, asking inwardly for Reiki's guidance, and practicing.

COMMUNITY SERVICE

We can develop our relationship with Reiki through self-treatment alone, but sometimes students feel a desire to offer Reiki to others.

Reiki has become so popular, respected, and trusted that many hospitals, hospices, nursing homes, and even schools are using volunteers to offer treatment. The requirements for volunteers vary among the venues and often include a general application process and volunteer training that are separate from the Reiki program. One usually need not be a professional practitioner to offer service. Professionalism, however, is always important.

If you become a Reiki volunteer, you will likely be asked to use an approved protocol when working on site even if it is different from how you practice at home. Hospitals, hospices, and other conventional care environments are understandably concerned that Reiki not look weird to patients, visitors, or medical staff, and usually frown on waving hands over the body, for example. When offering Reiki in any public capacity, it is important to maintain boundaries and not offer intuitive feedback or engage in conversation beyond introducing yourself.

If you choose to volunteer, be mindful to leave your service at the site. If you notice you're bringing it home with you, if you find yourself stewing about the people you treat or feel that your service is affecting your emotional well-being, take a careful look at what is happening inside. This inner hygiene is vital. Most volunteer work is done with people who are facing serious illness. They have enough on their plate without being burdened by their caregivers' unresolved emotions. The people we serve need and deserve to be cared for, honored, and empowered, not infantilized, pitied, and victimized—and they feel the difference. But enough about them: It's not healthy for you to be in a situation in which you can't hold your boundaries. Give yourself Reiki and contemplate what's happening.

BECOMING A REIKI PROFESSIONAL

Reiki training teaches you how to practice Reiki; it does not prepare you to be a Reiki professional. Of course, the most important foundation for becoming a professional is considerable practice, both daily self-treatment and giving or receiving treatment. Professionals also need skills in communication, clinical practice, and business. And, especially if you want to collaborate in medical settings, it is helpful to have an understanding of medical culture, professional standards, and research (see page 241). I offer in-person training, individual mentoring, and teleclasses to help Reiki practitioners prepare themselves for professional practice and health-care collaboration. (My travel schedule is at www.ReikiInMedicine.org.)

If you plan to become a Reiki professional, you might consider an unpaid internship that provides professional training and clinical experience. Make ample use of whatever supervision is available to you, both in the health-care facility and from your Reiki master, and ask your on-site supervisor for periodic service evaluations, as would be given to paid staff. If you are thinking of using your volunteer position as a stepping-stone to employment in the institution, find out ahead of time if that is possible. Some organizations preclude volunteers from transitioning to paid positions.

Creating and then maintaining discipline and routine may be the least intriguing aspect of developing a meaningful Reiki practice, but once you are initiated, it is the most important. It creates the foundation for everything your Reiki practice will bring. After all, what is Reiki practice but *practice*?

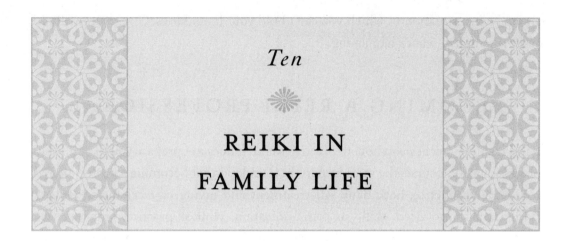

Ten

REIKI IN
FAMILY LIFE

Everybody is all right really.

A. A. MILNE, *WINNIE THE POOH*

Helen placed her hand on her four-year-old son's head at bedtime one night during her First Degree training. "Is this supposed to calm me down?" he asked. "Yes," she said. "Is it working?" "Yes," he answered.

The same adorable child made a halfhearted attempt to derail his parents' anniversary dinner plans by pointing out that he couldn't go to sleep because their babysitter can't give Reiki. He reconsidered when his mom promised Reiki when she got home, but only if he was asleep.

Reiki mommies not only have the usual eyes in back of our heads, we also have sensors in our hands. As I affectionately greeted my kids after school, Reiki occasionally alerted me that something needed attention. Whenever my hand activated during a welcome-home hug, gentle questioning elicited a tale of woe—a taunting, a disappointing test score, a cold coming on. My kids thought I was a magic mommy who could read their lives. Who was I to argue?

Takata encouraged her students to treat themselves first and then offer Reiki to family and friends. Let Reiki enter your family life gently and organically. Start with your own practice and let Reiki bubble over to the kids in time. Don't link Reiki to punishment or even to avoiding punishment. Let it be part of everyday life, a daily practice that can be used more often when needed. As a daily practice, Reiki fits easily with bedtime. Parents can offer their children a Reiki hand for a few minutes, or children who have been trained can practice on themselves—or both at the same time.

REIKI FOR PREGNANCY

I learned Reiki early in my last pregnancy, and the difference in my health and stamina was immediate. The wisdom and practicality of taking care of pregnant women is obvious. There is also increasing scientific evidence not only of the degree to which prenatal and maternal stress affects babies in utero and after birth, but also of how it happens. Chronic stress during pregnancy has been linked to sleeping and feeding problems after the baby is born, as well as anxiety, symptoms of attention-deficit hyperactivity disorder (ADHD), aggressiveness and behavioral problems as children grow.[1] In addition, research has traced the roots of heart disease, cancer, osteoporosis, and other conditions to the womb, in ways that are separate from genetic influences, although maternal behavior also alters genes.[2]

It is apparent that protecting a mother's well-being also protects her child's. Pregnancy is a time of uncertainty and constant change. Some women feel out of control, especially during the birthing process. Reiki—the "mother's milk" of subtle therapies—helps soothe both mother and baby.

Takata said it is best if the woman receives treatment before getting pregnant, after miscarriage, then during pregnancy to strengthen her, and more if any symptoms appear.[3] Wanja Twan remembers that when treating pregnant women, Takata often placed her hand directly on the heart, saying it was beating for two.

For many women, the exhaustion of late pregnancy leads to the most strenuous labor of their lives, with no time to recover afterward. Exhaustion deepens in the weeks (or months) before the baby settles into a sleep pattern. Reiki helps new moms relax quickly and sleep more deeply, even if they don't get to sleep for long.

REIKI AND CHILDREN

I was a Reiki mom long before I became a soccer mom. It was hard to watch kids get hurt on the field and not be able to use my Reiki hands to calm them and help lessen their pain and trauma in the moments right after injury. This was part of my motivation to start coaching. Coaches are supposed to go out to injured players, and although fortunately we had no serious injuries, Reiki's touch soothed many felled players. When my daughter's athletic skill exceeded mine and she graduated to a more experienced coach, he was surprised at how quickly her injuries healed. Reiki is quite literally a first-aid kit in the hand. With accidents being the main reason children under ten see their doctors, that's no small thing. And it's just one of the ways Reiki helps kids.

Offering Reiki to children requires a light touch, literally and figuratively. I've never had a child refuse treatment, but some are decidedly more interested than others. There is no need to be rigid in offering treatment to kids. Be mindful of the hand placements, follow the sensation in your hands, or just do what you can. With a baby, one hand on the head and/or one on the torso may be enough. Children typically respond faster than adults and need less treatment. Especially when treating children (including teens), we are wise to remember Takata's teaching: "Reiki will guide you. Let the Reiki hands find it. They will know what to do."

I have also seen good results training children with autism, Asperger's, and other developmental syndromes. The causes of autism are unknown, and much controversy surrounds it. Because Reiki is balancing, it can be of benefit regardless of the cause, and can provide soothing moments for parents and kids alike. Children who learn Reiki benefit from the empowerment as well as its centering effect. Practicing Reiki enrolls the family in a culture of wellness.

According to Lawrence Palevsky, M.D., FAAP, former chief of pediatric acute care at Lenox Hill Hospital in New York City, one of the biggest issues for kids today is maintaining acceptable behavior while dealing with anxieties, fears, emotions, peer pressures, and educational pressures. In addition, the range of childhood ailments— ear infections, respiratory infections, asthma, gastrointestinal upset—is extending to include many conditions that once plagued only adults, such as Type 2 (adult-onset) diabetes. Palevsky sees Reiki as a valuable part of care, one that can quietly address the emotional component of conditions such as asthma and irritable bowel syndrome while empowering kids with another tool for self-regulation.

At Lenox Hill, Palevsky was responsible for the care of children in the neonatal and pediatric intensive care unit (ICU). He routinely used Reiki to enhance medical outcomes for neonates. While carefully monitoring vital signs and administering oxygen if needed, Palevsky would place hands on the head and torso of a baby born in distress, flaccid, nonresponsive, weak, or not crying. Generally, within ten to fifteen minutes of Reiki, babies opened their eyes, moved around, and developed increasing body tone. No other medical intervention was needed.

Palevsky also gave Reiki to babies born suppressed from obstetrical interventions such as those involving forceps or extractions performed as a response to perceived fetal distress, or babies born with distress caused by complications such as cord around neck or prolonged labor. In cases when respiratory problems did not resolve or the baby's distress seemed to intensify, Palevsky would take appropriate medical intervention, continuing Reiki as possible in the neonatal intensive care unit (NICU). Reiki treatment did not interfere with needed medical care, and was continued until the baby's vital signs showed that no further intervention was needed. Palevsky followed all the babies until they went home.

Nearly all the babies who received Reiki avoided NICU admission. The babies who avoided intensive care had no further medical complications and went home in a timely manner. Although life-saving care is provided in the NICU, high-tech critical care brings its own discomforts and potential complications. Stabilizing a new-born and avoiding intensive care is good medicine.

Palevsky has also administered Reiki during nebulizer treatment for asthmatic children, infants, and adolescents in the ER, the ICU, the inpatient unit, and in his private medical office. He simultaneously offered breathing instructions. Some children with only mild wheezing responded to Reiki and breathing instructions and did not need the nebulizer. Palevsky's experience has convinced him that Reiki can safely minimize or avoid medications.

Sometimes physicians unfamiliar with Reiki express concern about using it with newborns. They fear that, as I've heard it, "the energy will overwhelm" the infant. This concern comes out of the medical model in which an intervention that helps also has the ability to harm. If we go back to the basics and remember that Reiki encourages balance and is precipitated by the recipient's need, it's apparent that Reiki is not dangerous at any age, or during pregnancy.

REIKI AND ADHD

Daniel decided to learn Reiki after seeing his ailing father improve from Reiki treatment. Daniel started class markedly skeptical—not of Reiki (he'd witnessed its benefit to his dad)—but of his ability to learn it. I was intrigued when he arrived for the second class bragging about his amazing son, an eleven-year-old boy diagnosed with ADHD. His son was at that wonderful and fleeting moment poised on the brink of being a full-fledged teen, yet still open to physical affection. Each night, Daniel would lie like a spoon with his son, to help him settle into sleep. One night, Daniel decided to give Reiki a try and lightly rested his hand on the crown of his son's head. Within moments, the boy said matter-of-factly, "Dad, your hand is vibrating."

Not yet confident about his own experience of Reiki, Daniel thought his son was precocious, and he well may be. But children notice subtle vibrations easily, and kids with attention-deficit disorder (ADD) or ADHD or learning disabilities seem especially aware in this area. Their distractability is related to their sensitivity. Imagine being a child so highly attuned to subtle reality, whose awareness is not valued at school, and who may have no adult around who can even validate that subtle awareness. These kids take readily to Reiki, and love the independence and empowerment it brings. I've seen Reiki help many kids come to a more harmonious relationship with themselves and the world around them.

REIKI AND TEENS

Reiki continues to benefit kids through the teen years, when the immediate relaxation and not having to talk about themselves are particularly appealing. So many teens struggle with self-regulation. Many truly gifted kids don't conform easily and have trouble finding their own rhythms. They are resistant to attempts to "fix" them, and who wouldn't be? I have seen kids who wouldn't accept other support melt on the Reiki table.

One adolescent I am particularly fond of completely baffled his parents. They didn't know what he wanted or needed. Our families knew each other, and he agreed to come for Reiki. During each treatment, he fell into a deep state within moments of lying on the table, his body twitching as the kinks in his nervous system unwound. His sense of relief was palpable as he started feeling at home in himself.

Lucky teens in Camden, Maine, have found Reiki at school. Camden Hills Regional High School is attended by 750 kids from five communities. According to Judy Ottman, M.Ed., the school lost eight students to a rash of accidents, drowning, and suicides within a six-month period in 2001. As part of the community's desire to support the teens through these tragedies, a Wellness Room was created to offer Reiki to students and staff. Students can come in on their own, or at the suggestion of a teacher or the school nurse. In the 2003–2004 school year, there were 370 student visits. Students lobbied to be trained themselves, and three Reiki masters collaborated to train twenty-four students in First Degree. A year later, eight of the student practitioners requested and received Second Degree training. A wide cross-section of students makes use of the Wellness Room. More than half the student body has received treatment, and the entire basketball team came in before an important game.

We needn't wait until teens show signs of stress to introduce them to Reiki as a way to center themselves and regain a sense of control. If Reiki is presented in a neutral setting, teens often feel drawn to experience it, and they appreciate the quick results Reiki can bring. Moreover, when a teen is troubled, Reiki can be a lifesaver, relieving suffering and alienation and opening the teen to receive support from other avenues. I have worked with teens and adults with anorexia and bulimia—two serious and resistant conditions—who used Reiki as part of a multifaceted, interdisciplinary treatment plan that enabled them to heal.

TRAINING CHILDREN TO PRACTICE REIKI

An eight-year-old student who's been practicing for three years told me, "Reiki has helped me in a lot of situations when I was really hurt. It calmed me down and made me feel better." His mom (one of my favorite cooks) was a little more forthcoming. Her son, she said, "is a bit of a hypochondriac. . . . The slightest bang or scratch makes him quite upset. So whenever he's been 'afflicted' he usually remembers that he can give himself Reiki, and he always feels as if it's much better after that. He's quite giving when it comes to others, too. There have been times (many times, I'm certain) when my clumsiness gets in the way and I have either sliced my fingers (cooking), burned myself (also cooking), or have just been careless (these are not always cooking-related). He always offers to give me Reiki, and he always wants to know if it's better."

In spite of all the evidence that life includes pain, our society persists in trying to protect children from feeling pain at all cost instead of equipping them with the spiritual skills to learn to be present with pain and learn from it. Addressing kids' emotional needs on a daily basis pays lifelong dividends. Use Reiki as a healing intervention when needed, but the best results come from introducing it as a practice. This could start as daily treatment by a parent, often at bedtime. At some point, the child can be trained as well. At what age? According to Reiki master Wanja Twan, Takata trained kids at age four.

I don't have an age cutoff for training kids, but rather evaluate each situation as it occurs. I especially look to see that the child wants to learn Reiki, that it's not just the parent's idea. If an entire family is practicing and one child is quite young, but willing, it may not make sense to exclude him.

It seems unwise to initiate younger children unless a parent is practicing Reiki. As kids develop, they need the support of a parent who is in touch with healing. This need fades as adolescents become more self-directed and have more freedom. A teen who encounters Reiki outside the home likely has some other support system through which he encountered it. But I always ask for parental permission when training teens who come to me without a parent.

Kids' classes are best geared to the ages and personalities of the students. Kids really just need the initiations and some basic instructions. Wanja Twan, mother of four and grandmother of seven, says, "We don't want Reiki to interfere with the kids' lives. The initiations will have their effect over the years." Wanja has repeatedly seen how kids respond after receiving treatment. She says, "They feel in their bodies that this is something they didn't know existed. It gives them hope for the future. It makes life more exciting to live."

Yo'el Erez is the son of two Reiki masters, Amy and Ofer, who have been masters since before he was born. As you can imagine, Yo'el has received a lot of Reiki in his life, but his parents did not rush to initiate him. Rather, they waited for him to feel and express the desire to be initiated, and to maintain that desire for a period of time. At age five, Yo'el began asking to be initiated. Six months later, a class was arranged. Around age nine, Yo'el realized he didn't know very much about pain, since Reiki was always available to balance any trauma. He refused treatment for several months, allowing himself to feel the pain that accompanies life's bumps and bruises. This gave him the experience to recognize what needed treatment and what was simply daily life. Twelve and a half at the time of this writing, Yo'el continues to give himself treatment as needed and ask for it when he wants.

REIKI, PARENTS, AND CHILDREN

Parents have full authority to make treatment decisions for their children, but a child can choose to learn Reiki, or not. We can't force anyone to heal, not even a child. We can offer opportunities, and we can model healing. Kids are more likely to want to learn Reiki if it has been in their environment and not been forced on them, and if they are left to use it as they choose. Kids learn a lot when they see parents make self-treatment a priority. Think of the flight attendant's instructions on your last plane trip. If the oxygen mask comes down, we're told to put it on ourselves first, then on our dependents. Our kids depend on us to take care of ourselves so we can take care of them.

As parents, we can't help wanting to protect our children from every possible harm. Of course, it's not possible to do that. What we can do is imbue our children with the confidence that they can address anything life brings their way. We are best equipped to do this by addressing our own anxieties for their safety because we are not able to control their lives and it's not healthy for us to try—not healthy for us and not healthy for them.

My prescription for parental anxiety? Reiki treatment once a day and more as needed, for the children, sure, but especially for the parents. To a great extent, we are the context in which our children live. We may actually impact our kids' well-being even more through regular self-treatment than we can through treating them directly. The steadier we are, the more we model wellness for our children, and the more easily we connect with our inner knowing even in times of fear.

REIKI AND OUR CHILDREN'S FUTURE HEALTH

Much of adult health is created in childhood, both on an emotional level and on very physical levels that may or may not be related to injuries. For example, a study showed that girls who sustain soccer injuries to their knees have a higher chance of developing a potentially disabling arthritis when they're older.[4] (It's possible there is an as-yet unrecognized underlying condition, perhaps a constitutional weakness, that predisposes some people to both injury and arthritis.)

According to traditional, holistic medical systems, such underlying differences explain why some kids (and adults) incline toward asthma or food allergies while others are vulnerable to panic attacks or learning irregularities. Although biomedical research gives some indications of underlying conditions, this is not yet well understood in conventional medicine. Meanwhile we know that kids are being impacted by stresses that shape their well-being now and in the future.

With Reiki, we don't have to know all the details to be taking an effective step toward maintaining our children's well-being. By helping kids to regain balance, Reiki can strengthen their bodies' self-regulatory mechanisms and help prevent or minimize a wide range of problems, physically, mentally, and emotionally, without risk to natural pediatric development or concern about side effects. Being able to reduce stress and reconnect with a sense of wellness every day might help reduce the risk of diabetes, arthritis, asthma, and food sensitivities. Reiki can take a lot of the guesswork out of maintaining your kids' optimal health.

REIKI AND SELF-ESTEEM

Concerns about self-esteem and social isolation that are felt in childhood recur throughout our lives. Richard Davidson's research on adult meditators has shown that the meditators had decreased activity in the part of the brain associated with negative emotion.[5] The implication is that meditators are more likely to frame life in a positive way. Although it has not yet been studied, it is feasible that Reiki offers at least some of the benefits of meditation, perhaps helping to develop the neural circuitry that supports equanimity and enables kids of all ages to better manage negative feelings, or even to have fewer. What horizons are being opened for children who have Reiki's ability to balance at their fingertips and who grow up with the reality of Reiki, aware of the continuum of matter and spirit? How might growing up with a pragmatic relationship with the unseen shape a child's understanding of the world? What impact might that have on the pandemic of postmodern alienation and isolation?

At six years of age, after practicing Reiki for six months, Yo'el Erez wrote this poem, which was published in *Reiki Magazine International:*[6]

God is willing
Deep inside
Give me the face
Of myself.

REIKI AND SENIORS

As the details of our families continually change, Reiki remains a constant companion, as relevant to Grandma's aches and pains as to her granddaughter's soccer injuries, and something they enjoy together. One of my older students returned for a Reiki reunion and gleefully announced, "There are three things I do every day: prayers, flossing, and Reiki. My soul is intact, I still have my teeth, and I no longer walk with a cane." Another senior spoke of using Reiki preventively when she's running late and thinks she might become anxious. "I'm going to be late is just an idea that doesn't have to become a reality," she said. "I practice Reiki and anxiety can be just another idea that doesn't become a reality."

Depending on their background, seniors may not have a conceptual context for Reiki, but it quickly doesn't matter to them. They've lived long enough to know when something feels good, they're pragmatic enough to grab onto it, and they're grateful it doesn't involve yet another medication. At a time when they need more and more assistance from others, seniors are enthusiastic to learn something they can do for themselves, even if they can't get out of bed.

Reiki helps seniors soothe anxiety, relieve pain, and sleep better. The Reiki circle or class where they learn creates a new and comfortable social environment for well-being. Many find Reiki helps them with side effects of medications.

Marjorie came to Reiki class in her mid-eighties. She was vague about her reasons, and I didn't pry. Her sincerity and commitment were apparent. After practicing for six months, she explained how debilitated by anxiety she had been, how she had "lost three years of my life to anxiety." Marjorie had exceptionally caring, competent physicians, but neither the cardiologist nor the psychopharmacologist could find medications that consistently worked well for her.

Although Marjorie did not have strong experiences while practicing Reiki, the difference in her well-being once she began Reiki self-treatment was dramatic. Within a month, she took a train by herself to visit family in the country. Her niece thanks Reiki for getting her favorite aunt out of her nightgown and out of the house. Marjorie noticed that if she drifted off while practicing in the late afternoon, she felt refreshed when she got up but was still able to fall asleep at her usual time and sleep well.

Depression in seniors is more prevalent than commonly realized even by family members and physicians.[7] It is associated with conditions that occur more frequently among seniors, such as Parkinson's disease, cancer, seizure disorder, diabetes, chronic lung disease, stroke, heart disease, severe pain, and with treatment for multiple diseases common in geriatric medicine. Depressed elders require greater assistance from others.[8] Seniors are at the highest risk of suicide of all Americans, with elderly men at greatest risk.[9] Suicide kills almost as many Americans aged sixty-five to seventy-four as does Alzheimer's disease. This is not a pattern seen across cultures.

Medical care becomes more complex as we age, and the failings of our current healthcare system falls hard on our senior population. Maximizing care while minimizing pharmaceuticals is always good medicine, but it is of particular concern with seniors. The body's ability to metabolize and excrete drugs weakens with age. The more medications a senior takes, the greater the risk of hazardous drug interactions. Some medications bring side effects that require still more medications. Seniors often find Reiki helps with side effects and many seniors using Reiki are able to reduce medications for anxiety or pain, under their doctors' supervision.

An illness or injury that requires a senior to be hospitalized often leads to permanent disability.[10] In my clinical experience, I've seen Reiki help shorten recovery time, enabling seniors to regain mobility faster and decreasing the likelihood of lasting disability. Additionally, there is emerging evidence that lifestyle changes can make a difference in a wide range of ailments that afflict seniors, such as Alzheimer's disease and hypertension. Strengthening well-being increases emotional and physical resilience.

DOROT, Inc., a senior outreach community center on the Upper West Side of Manhattan, launched a Reiki program in 1999. Karen Fuller, N.D., C.S.W., L.Ac., director of health and nutrition services, had invited me to introduce Reiki to the community and staff as part of a wellness-day menu the year before, and it was well received. Encouraged by the clients' enthusiasm, we offered classes and started an ongoing Reiki circle where students could meet to share treatment and others could stop by for a sample. When we learned that one of DOROT's clients was a Reiki master, I turned the group over to her.

There is no one modality that meets everyone's needs all the time. People are comfortable receiving in different ways. Offering a range of options is an important part of serving a community. The Reiki gatherings were another way DOROT could introduce healing and community support to its clients. Fuller commented that the Reiki circle provided a nucleus of support for people whose needs might not get addressed in other ways, offering hope, relaxation, reassurance, in a way that was very meaningful to the participants. "Reiki is an empowering modality," Fuller said.

Here's what some DOROT seniors told me about their Reiki experience:

"I feel calmer."
"I feel it's good and something I can accept."

"It's been a difficult two weeks. One night, after doing my Reiki, I felt that everything is okay."

"When I do Reiki, I begin to meditate. It's very reassuring."

"Each part of my body gets warm and feels alive."

"I feel more calm. I'm able to sleep better."

"It's nice to feel I have it as an ally. It helps me cope."

"It has an impact on many things."

"There was a family situation in which I became angry at my granddaughter. I wanted to teach her something about the way she was treating her mother, who is seriously ill, but I didn't want to speak out of anger. I gave myself Reiki and suddenly realized I wasn't feeling angry anymore. I felt sad. Finally I relaxed and understood a way I could talk to my granddaughter. When we did speak, it worked out very well."

Reiki groups in assisted-living facilities could engage seniors in doing something healthy for themselves. Seniors often feel isolated in their new environment even when they choose to move. The bonding aspect of Reiki could help seniors socialize and adjust to their changed circumstances. Reiki lifts seniors above the many indignities of growing old in America, helping them to truly age with grace.

REIKI, PAIN, AND PALLIATIVE CARE

None of us wants to be thought of as a hypochondriac. That said, it's important to address pain. Not just the cause of the pain—although that's also important—but the pain itself. Experiencing pain is stressful, and stress intensifies pain. Am I saying that your pain is all in your head? Not at all. If you feel it, it's real. And it may already be affecting your quality of life and that of your family. Why not explore how to relieve it?

Sometimes people don't want to get any help until they have a medical diagnosis. When it comes to Reiki treatment, this is not a concern. Reiki does not artificially mask pain (or any other symptom). By bringing you some relief, it may actually make your doctor's job easier. So yes, go to your doctor, but also try Reiki.

Palliative care is the medical specialty devoted to treating pain. Pain can be connected to an illness or an injury, or it may occur for reasons that conventional medicine cannot diagnose. In that case, pain itself is treated as a disease.

Many pain patients want to take as little medication as possible, and some just don't get much relief from medications, or the relief comes with troublesome side effects. Reiki can help (research evidence of this is discussed in chapter 13). We don't need to know the source of pain in order to feel relief from Reiki. Relief is usually felt during the first treatment, often within minutes, but the best results come with continued treatment over time, either self-treatment or treatment received from someone else, or both. Place a Reiki hand on the site of pain if that feels good to the patient, but to create the deepest healing possible, be sure to give a complete treatment.

Reiki can relieve pain associated with serious illness, even pain as intense as that accompanying sickle cell anemia. The Pain and Palliative Care Service of the National Institutes of Health's Warren Grant Magnuson Clinical Center in Bethesda, Maryland, where all patients enrolled in NIH clinical trials receive their medical care, includes Reiki as part of a broad palette of conventional and complementary techniques to treat suffering in people of all ages, patients as well as their families and loved ones. Suffering involves many forms of pain, including anxiety, social alienation, and psychospiritual distress, all of which respond readily to Reiki treatment. One of Reiki's greatest advantages is that anyone who is interested—children and other family, close friends, even the patient—can learn to practice.

Landis Vance, a chaplain and Reiki master at NIH Clinical Center, sometimes teaches Reiki to patients and families. She notes that being able to relieve the suffering of someone they love keeps family members from feeling helpless and engaging in futile, sometimes irritating activity, such as constantly plumping pillows. Having Reiki hands available to them can ease the burden of those who are suffering and create powerful moments of bonding. Especially if the patient is included, training should be tailored to the immediate situation. If needed, the conceptual aspects of training may be left aside as family members participate in sharing Reiki with one another.

REIKI AND DYING

Dying is part of living and of family life, a passage for which we are too often ill prepared. It is natural for families to draw together when a family member is dying. Reiki can support the person who is dying and also loved ones by relieving the physical, emotional, and spiritual pain experienced at the end of life. Reiki's effectiveness in end-of-life care is quickly noticed by hospice professionals, and many hospices now include Reiki. Whether your loved one is receiving hospice support at home or is in a residential facility, inquire if any of the hospice staff is Reiki-trained.

Reiki provides a quiet activity that family members can engage in together as they choose, bonding even more deeply as they support one another. Sometimes everyone, including the dying person and children, gathers for a family training. It is not necessary for everyone to be involved, however, and one should not pressure reluctant family members. The presence of even a single Reiki practitioner in the family can be a source of support to all, including those who may not want to receive treatment directly. The profound comfort Reiki brings to the dying is obvious, and that alone is an enormous relief.

Sometimes I am called to give treatment to someone who is dying. During these visits, I offer a few minutes of chair Reiki to any family member who is interested. Reiki silently connects each person to her own unique spirituality, easing her passage through this profoundly spiritual time.

Children are often overlooked when a family member is dying, either because of the demands of the time or in an attempt to shield them from pain. Even young children can participate in Reiki. It gives them a way to address their own anxiety and sadness that they instinctively understand and enables them to connect with and contribute to the patient and other family members.

Reiki Can Reduce the Need for Pain Medication

It's important that pain be managed in a way that is medically sound and agreeable to the patient. Many patients who want to be pain-free also want to maintain clarity of mind through the dying process. Although I always encourage clients to take their pain medication as needed, many patients, even with metastatic cancer, remain pain-free using Reiki and minimal medication, and sometimes only Reiki. Perhaps this is because Reiki relieves the emotional and spiritual problems that are so elusive yet greatly compound pain. Not only does Reiki reduce pain, it also brings profound peace and remarkable clarity.

People at the end of life may face other discomforts besides pain, such as breathlessness that may not be related to lack of oxygen. Reiki often makes breathing more comfortable, and it can relieve overall tension and nausea caused by disease or medications. The benefits of Reiki treatment vary from patient to patient, and they can be long-lasting. Offer as much Reiki as is comfortable for the patient and the practitioner. Reiki can be given to someone who is asleep or unconscious.

Weariness and loss of appetite are common symptoms as a person approaches death. It can be difficult for families to accept that more food or even better-quality food will not return their loved one to health. The desire to nourish a failing loved one is deep-seated in our hearts. Reiki offers the spiritual nourishment needed by the patient and helps everyone connect with the timeliness of dying. It restores a sense of balance even amid the experience of loss. The serenity that can come from Reiki treatment is unmistakable.

REIKI AND ANIMALS

I wish all my students were as enthusiastic about self-treatment as pet owners are about treating their animals. One effusive student named her new kittens Hawayo and Takata. Another loves giving Reiki to her turtle. She feels Reiki pulsing in her hands as she holds her beloved pet, and senses that it settles him. Even when he's been startled, he'll settle down in her hands, gradually releasing his limbs and head out of his shell.

Animals are very aware of the change that occurs in their owners' presence when they start practicing Reiki. The night after her first initiation, a psychotherapist's Siamese cats purred so loudly that even her husband noticed. They vied for position, with one always at her feet and the other on her lap. Most animals like Reiki, although occasionally I hear of one who is indifferent to it.

Being with nature in any form raises our awareness of Reiki. For city dwellers, animals are a concentrated dose of nature. If you have an opportunity to offer Reiki to an animal, try it and see how it compares to treating adult humans! Animals (and children) are not talking themselves out of their experience. If they like it, they stay put. If they've had enough, they get up and leave.

Maggie was very conflicted over what to do for her cat, a beloved companion of sixteen years who was nearing death. Although Reiki relieved his pain and distress, and the peace Reiki brought both of them was undeniable, Maggie feared it wouldn't be enough and she didn't want her cat to suffer. Although I never expressed an opinion, our conversations about Reiki brought Maggie the support she needed to trust her heart. Her cat died peacefully with her Reiki hands on him. She thanked Reiki for enabling them to be together as nature took its course, which she preferred to taking him to the vet.

"As soon as I started putting my hands on horses professionally, it was pretty amazing," says Woodstock, New York, Reiki master Cindy Brody. "The owners didn't particularly believe in what I was doing but once they saw the difference Reiki made, they didn't care about their beliefs." Brody is the owner of CinergE, a service that provides equine energy balancing, bodywork, Reiki, and animal communication.

Most of the horses Brody works with have been in her care for six or seven years. She treats them once a month. Her equine clients earn a lot of ribbons and rarely get injured, which she attributes to their being in good health and being centered. The horses are happy and the owners are happy, she says. Brody may be the only Reiki practitioner whose clients have been "referred" by horses.

Reiki master Elena Jespersen gives all her horses a weekly treatment. Jesperson's horses particularly like Reiki at the front of the face and between the ears. While receiving Reiki, her horses often hang their heads and sleep like people in a Reiki slumber. Jesperson says, "Horses are like cats and dogs in that they'll walk off when they're finished." Jesperson has worked with colic and many lameness injuries and says Reiki helps her horses heal faster. Giving Reiki to the neck while walking a colicky horse, she sees a rapid and noticeable lessening of pain and overall relaxation. She says, "Reiki calms the horse's mind and relaxes the gut." One of Jesperson's foals had a broken leg. After daily treatment for a couple of weeks, X-rays showed complete recovery, and he grew to be a rideable horse.

One of the many joys of Reiki is sharing it. While it is most important to treat yourself first and ensure your own well-being and balance, sharing Reiki with those you love—family members, friends, even beloved pets—will deepen and expand your relationship with Reiki.

Eleven

REIKI, DOCTORS, AND PATIENTS

*The doctor of the future will give no medication, but will interest his patients
in the care of the human frame, diet, and in the cause and prevention of disease.*

THOMAS A. EDISON

A family doctor at an inner-city clinic offers to hold his eighty-three-year-old patient's aching hand while they talk about her health. Although he is focused on his patient, he notices Reiki sensations softly pulsing in his hands throughout their conversation. The next day, she leaves a message saying both hands feel better. What made the difference? Reiki or placebo? Or simply the touch of a caring human being and physician? Does it matter? Patient and doctor were happy with the interaction and the result. What more could we want from health care?

The Harvard team that studied how Americans were using complementary and alternative medicine (CAM) in the 1990s stunned the medical establishment with their results. The researchers found that a startling percentage of the population was already using CAM, a much higher number than conventional doctors imagined. The research team also discovered that patients were paying out-of-pocket for these services—laying out more cash, in fact, than they were for their conventional medical care. But Americans were not forsaking conventional care for CAM; they were using both.[1]

Patients were not, however, telling their physicians what they were doing. By not telling their physicians, they were essentially taking control of their health care away from their doctors. This concerns physicians, and with reason; certain CAM therapies and products can affect conventional medical interventions, not the least of which is potential drug-herb interactions. But none of that is a concern with Reiki, because the touch is nonmanipulative and there is nothing ingested that could interfere with medications. If you quit smoking or drinking caffeine or took up meditation hoping to improve your health, you would probably tell your doctor. Why not mention Reiki?

SPEAKING TO YOUR PHYSICIAN ABOUT REIKI

The mere thought of telling your physician that you've been practicing Reiki, or even bringing the subject up, may make you uncomfortable. What if your doctor makes fun of you? (It happens.) She may more than pooh-pooh your efforts to heal yourself; she may put the kibosh on it. After all, physicians are trained in medical science to work with phenomena they can observe, measure, and treat. Moreover, given the time pressures of today's doctor visits due to high costs and managed care, you may not want to waste any of your seven-minute appointment on something you don't expect your doctor even to know about. You may not want to risk your relationship with your physician; if she is negative about something that's important to you, it might affect your care. But are you sure that hiding it from her isn't already affecting your relationship?

If you think of your doctor as your partner in health care, there are many reasons to build a good, honest relationship. You may want to know sooner rather than later how he defines his role in your care, how open-minded and collaborative he is. It makes sense for everyone on your care team to know about everyone else, even if they are not in direct communication. It gives you confidence to know that all the members of your health-care team support what you are doing with the other team members.

Doctors are usually interested in what helps their patients without causing harm. I know many doctors who have been impressed by an improvement in symptoms and overall well-being that their patient attributes to Reiki. Some have gone on to tell other patients about Reiki, or even to learn it themselves. Most doctors caring for patients understand it takes more than science to create well-being. If you've found something that helps you and that is not dangerous, why wouldn't your doctor support it? If he doesn't, you may determine that you and your physician are not philosophically compatible and you might consider looking elsewhere for care.

Although it is not dangerous to use Reiki if you are on medication—again, there is nothing about Reiki that interacts with the drugs—Reiki may help you heal in ways that affect your need for medication. For example, although I haven't worked with many diabetics, the ones I have worked with who needed insulin experienced a reduced need for it when using Reiki regularly. This is only anecdotal evidence— that is, based on reports of individual cases—but it has been the case both for people to whom I have given Reiki treatment and for those I have taught to practice Reiki self-treatment.

Similarly, people I have worked with who take pain medication on an as-needed basis have needed less—or even none—once they started receiving Reiki treatment or giving themselves Reiki. If you are on medication—especially for pain, depression, anxiety, insomnia, diabetes or hormonal imbalances, side effects of other medications, or even hypertension—speak to your doctor about the possibility that you might need less medication once you start Reiki treatment. Find out how to monitor your need and be sure you understand what to watch for. Physicians generally agree that it is best to use the lowest effective dose of medication and will be pleased if you are able to reduce your prescriptions. However, it's important that your physician supervise this transition. Some drugs cause withdrawal symptoms or a disease flare if they are stopped abruptly.

SPEAKING TO YOUR DOCTOR— BE PREPARED

Why not give your doctor a chance to surprise you? If you're using Reiki, why not educate your doctor about it, and if you're not, she might educate you, or you might learn together. If you don't mention it, you'll never know. I know physicians who are supportive of complementary therapies—Reiki and others—but only mention them to patients who start the conversation. There is no way to identify these doctors from the outside, and some of the most scientifically oriented physicians turn out be the most open-minded about using an "unproven" therapy if there is no evidence that it will harm you. When I give hospital grand rounds, there are all kinds of doctors and medical professionals there, men and women of varying ages and experience, and no one has yet thrown a tomato at me. Maybe your doctor heard a similar presentation just last week.

But maybe she didn't. Be prepared in case your physician doesn't know anything about Reiki, and don't assume this is a negative. This is your opportunity. Make the best of it. Put together a few sentences that express Reiki—not explain it. Be sure to communicate why Reiki is important to you. A lot depends on the way you express yourself, and whether you let your doctor know up-front that Reiki is not dangerous, and that Reiki supports the work you do together, rather than supplanting it. Be clear to yourself that you are informing your physician of a choice you have made, not asking for permission. Doctors are concerned about accountability.

Here are the points your doctor will want to know:

- Reiki is balancing to the recipient.
- There are no known medical contraindications—Reiki is never dangerous.
- The touch is light; there is no pressure or manipulation.
- There is no substance to ingest, so there is nothing to interact with medications.
- Reiki safely combines with and supports any medical intervention, including surgery, medications, radiation or chemotherapy, and physical therapy.

- Reiki is calming and refreshing (if you are already using Reiki, list the ways in which you benefit from treatment and express how important it is to you).

Bring some Reiki literature you can leave with your doctor. Perhaps your practitioner has a brochure, or print out something from my website (www.ReikiInMedicine.org), or refer her directly to the website. It was created with physicians in mind and has medical papers written in language that is meaningful to them (some articles have been translated into other languages). The website also has articles detailing how Reiki is being used in hospitals, including the Clinical Center of the National Institutes of Health (NIH) in Bethesda, Maryland. Give your doctor the information she needs to support your choice. If she isn't supportive, ask what her concern is. If you don't know how to address it, let her know you'll do some research and get back to her. Making it a priority to do so promptly shows her that this is important to you.

WHO BENEFITS FROM REIKI?

Physicians unfamiliar with Reiki often want to know which of their patients might benefit. I asked a student of mine, Danna Park, M.D., FAAP, who practices integrative medicine and is a clinical assistant professor in the Program in Integrative Medicine at the University of Arizona. She replied, "This is kind of a trick question because anyone could benefit from Reiki, and I can't imagine anyone not benefiting." Park understands that because Reiki is balancing, it can help anyone. But that doesn't mean that every patient will gravitate toward Reiki, so I asked Park how she decides when she will suggest Reiki to a patient.

I think of Reiki for people who are dealing with a lot of stress and who are real go-getters, doing, doing, doing, always doing. Reiki is a way to receive and not have to do. Reiki is also useful for those who have had a lot of chronic body issues and who don't feel connected to their bodies or who feel frustrated by their bodies, such as patients with fibromyalgia or arthritis. Anyone who has used mind/body medicine will also appreciate Reiki because it helps bring their awareness inward.

New York City internist Michael Gnatt is likely to offer Reiki to patients who are "tense, wired, stressed out or upset." Sometimes he offers a full Reiki treatment, or more often, he'll use Reiki during a physical exam. When examining a tense abdomen, for example, he rests his hand lightly on the abdomen until he feels the patient's muscles relax, allowing a more comfortable exam. A referral for Reiki training or treatment may naturally unfold from that experience, or he may simply continue with the physical.

When assessing a patient for Reiki, Ann Berger, M.D., head of the Pain and Palliative Care Service at the NIH Clinical Center in Bethesda, Maryland, looks not at the diagnosis but at the patient's overall state. She recommends Reiki for patients with "pain and anxiety, and the spiritual suffering that often manifests as pain and anxiety." She notes that Reiki is useful especially for patients who are not verbally expressive, supporting their ability and willingness to articulate their needs.

When people are very ill, telling them how much they need to change their lifestyle to support their well-being might plunge them into feelings of hopelessness. Doctors can give their patients a little Reiki and suggest further treatment or training. Reiki will quickly impact patients' sense of self-agency. With an improved outlook and functioning, patients can then hear what else has to be done. Reiki is a logical and effective first step that creates a strong foundation for healing.

REIKI IN THE HOSPITAL

You might want to have a Reiki practitioner accompany you during a medical procedure, birth, or surgery. If the Reiki practitioner is also a licensed medical professional, there shouldn't be any problem, even in surgery. If not, you may have to compromise. If the surgeon or physician is supportive, it may be possible to have a Reiki practitioner in the operating room. (I have offered Reiki in the OR, including during heart transplantation.) It is important that the practitioner know how to conduct himself in that environment. If you can't work out the details to get your Reiki practitioner into the OR, your doctor will likely compromise by getting him into the recovery room to treat you. (Family members are usually brought into recovery at some point). Ask your surgeon for permission for your Reiki practitioner to stay with you longer than is usually allowed. Navigating medical turf calls for a deft combination of deference, diplomacy, and confidence. So much of what happens in recovery or the intensive care unit (ICU) depends on the attitude of the nurse assigned to that patient. If your Reiki practitioner has not worked in this situation before, coach him in the importance of being collaborative and respectful of what the medical team is doing. If the Reiki practitioner lets the nurse do her job, the nurse will likely let the practitioner do his. The Reiki practitioner can always step aside to get out of the nurse's way. It's never a problem to interrupt a Reiki treatment, and in the hospital, the practitioner is generally using a modified Reiki treatment plan anyway, working around wires and tubes, treating patients who often can't be turned.

On the other hand, the practitioner may have to gently and diplomatically stand his ground and remind the nurse that he is there at the request of the patient and with the surgeon's permission. But be aware that if the Reiki practitioner handles the situation poorly, it is unlikely the next request will be granted.

Make sure you're clear about what the arrangements are. One client who wanted me to attend her birth told the hospital (unbeknownst to me) that I was a doula (a birthing coach). There was an awkward moment when the obstetrician told me to get the patient ready to push. Fortunately, she didn't have time to push. We all laughed about it later, and the physician was impressed by how Reiki helped his anxious patient maintain a relatively calm demeanor.

Hospital Reiki Programs

Reiki programs are sprouting up in hospitals like well-germinated seeds. Portsmouth Regional Hospital in Portsmouth, New Hampshire, has the largest and longest-running Reiki program I have come across. Started in 1995 by Patricia Alandydy, R.N., Portsmouth gives more than two thousand Reiki sessions each year to patients in all parts of the hospital. There is a full-time lay Reiki master on paid staff. A well-screened and -trained volunteer corps covers the hospital when she is not available so that patients can access Reiki seven days a week. Patients are referred to Reiki by physicians, nurses, or other medical staff, or by family members. Many patients read the Reiki notice that is in each hospital room and request treatment on their own. The hospital created a "Reiki Satisfaction Survey" that is used to evaluate the program on a quarterly basis.

The Warren Grant Magnuson Clinical Center of the National Institutes of Health in Bethesda is where patients enrolled in NIH clinical trials receive their medical care. Patients from all over the world who are fighting a wide range of conditions come there for treatment. The Clinical Center's Pain and Palliative Care Service (PPCS) offers state-of-the-art treatment to ease the suffering of these patients. It does so through the skilled use of both conventional and complementary modalities. Reiki is one of the complementary therapies used. The service at NIH was created by Ann Berger, M.D., who says, "We can't tell scientifically how it works, but it works. It somehow allows patients to heal inside without having long discussions with spiritual ministry." All PPCS therapies are integrated into medical care and may also be used in combination with other therapies. For example, a patient with a severe movement disorder (somewhat like Parkinson's disease) had some relief from hypnosis, but when Reiki was added, the improvement was much greater (and caught on film). Some staff have been trained, and patients who are receiving treatment over a period of time are sometimes initiated and trained in self-treatment.

In 2005, a partnership between the Institute for the Advancement of Complementary Therapies (I*ACT), a nonprofit organization I created to provide information and education to health-care practitioners and the general public and to foster research on complementary therapies, and St. Vincent's Comprehensive Care Center in New York City developed a program offering Reiki to patients, family members, and staff. Reiki can support cancer patients at every stage of treatment.[2] New patients and their family members experience relief from the anxiety a cancer diagnosis brings; patients in treatment comment that Reiki is restorative and reassuring, imparting a calmness and peacefulness. And after treatment is complete, Reiki helps patients regain the physical and emotional strength needed to return to a normal schedule, in the shadow of uncertainty regarding recurrence. Grazia Della-Terza offers Reiki to patients at St. Vincent's. She likens being a cancer patient to traveling in an overcrowded bus on a bumpy road, holding on white-knuckled just to get to the next stop. She says Reiki smooths the road.

Della-Terza affectionately coined the term "post-Reiki syndrome" to describe the hugging that goes on after treatment. In her experience as a bodyworker, hugs after a session were rare, and when they happened, often felt like the client's expression of emotional neediness. Della-Terza feels no neediness in post-Reiki hugs, just a sense of joy and celebration.

Many physicians have shared how moments of Reiki during an exam helped patients open up and start giving information, even of suicidal thoughts, that was critical to the patients' getting the needed care. This has happened even in clinics where physicians have only limited time to spend with patients.

HOW MEDICAL PROFESSIONALS ARE HELPING PATIENTS WITH REIKI

The infusion of Reiki into medicine goes far beyond dedicated programs. Medical professionals of all specialties are learning Reiki and incorporating it into routine care. Indeed, once you are Reiki-trained, Reiki can activate with any touch. Reiki requires no conscious intention, so it can pulse while the attention of caregivers is focused on the practice of medicine. The following are stories of how medical professionals I've trained are using Reiki with their patients.

Reiki and Pain

James Dillard, M.D., a pain specialist and the author of *The Chronic Pain Solution,* says, "Pain patients are often very flustered and going in many directions at once. There's a lot of anguish and frustration. Giving them Reiki quiets and calms them tremendously." Dillard finds Reiki helps with nausea and adverse reactions to pharmaceuticals, yet he finds the centering aspect most valuable in his practice. "Pain has a large emotional component, and Reiki is a very powerful tool for addrssing that," he observes. "It simplifies and stills patients, brings them back to their essence."

Reiki and Cancer Surgery

Bert M. Petersen, Jr., M.D., chief of breast surgery and co–division chief of breast oncology at Hackensack University Medical Center in New Jersey, trained in Reiki with me in 1998. Afterward, he started holding his patients' hands in the OR to offer Reiki while anesthesia was administered. The anesthesiologists he worked with soon began commenting how smoothly his patients went under. Petersen noticed that many patients were reluctant to take pain medication after surgery. At first he insisted, but when the patients who took pain medication in spite of their inclination not to do so often complained of nausea and/or feeling out of it, Petersen stopped insisting. Once they are at home after surgery, his patients frequently call to tell him how well they are feeling and how quickly they're recovering. He notes that postoperative visits are no longer taken up with pain concerns. Now there is time to address quality-of-life concerns such as fear of disfigurement and reduced functioning; this good doctor sees this time as a Reiki-given boon to his medical practice. One of this patients, herself a Reiki practitioner, felt something familiar coming from some of the pairs of hands prepping her for surgery. She surprised Petersen by asking, "Who's giving me Reiki?" She was equally surprised, and delighted, to learn that it was her surgeon.

Reiki Relieves Patients' Distress During Medical Intervention

Lewis Mehl-Madrona, M.D., Ph.D., found Reiki helpful during a study that required intravenous medication to be administered to autistic children, tots to teens. Insertion of the IV was problematic. The kids wouldn't cooperate until a nurse gave them individual Reiki treatments. Twenty minutes into the treatments, while the nurse continued offering Reiki, the doctor quietly entered the room and quickly inserted the IVs. The kids barely noticed.

Pat Toney, R.N., works at St. Vincent's Comprehensive Cancer Care Center in New York City. She assists during bone marrow biopsies, probably the most invasive medical procedure done with only local anesthesia. Toney keeps a Reiki hand on the patient's back during the procedure and receives grateful feedback. Patients find it calming and relaxing, and comment on how the gentle warmth of her hand draws their attention out of their anxiety. When they return, patients proudly introduce her to their family as the Reiki nurse.

Reiki Supports the Doctor-Patient Relationship

All doctors encounter challenging patients from time to time. When George Kessler, D.O., feels his interaction with a patient isn't going well, he'll suggest they try something different. Placing hands on the patient's head for a minute or two relaxes them both and opens a more fruitful conversation. One incredulous patient asked, "Are you giving me Reiki, Doctor?"

Reiki Can Help Even When Nothing Else Can Be Done

Several physicians have shared stories of how Reiki has supported their patients at those difficult times when medicine has nothing else to offer. The following anecdotes are particularly descriptive of the benefits Reiki offers both physician and patient.

Elena Klimenko, M.D., is a family-practice physician in an inner-city clinic. I taught her Reiki as part of the Integrative Medicine Fellowship Program at the Continuum Center for Health and Healing in New York City. One of Klimenko's patients was particularly troubling because of the complexity of her medical condition and the intensity of her suffering. The patient, a woman in her mid-thirties, was diagnosed with bipolar disorder and severe general anxiety disorder. She was also morbidly obese and a borderline diabetic with a seizure disorder. Klimenko decided to give a Reiki treatment during their appointment. For twenty minutes both doctor and patient relaxed deeply, and the patient left content and relieved of pain. Two weeks later, the patient arrived for her next visit without any prompting. Instead of the usual and understandable litany of complaints, she simply said, "I feel great." Although the medical problems were not solved, Klimenko knew this pronounced difference in her patient's sense of well-being and overall functioning was an important step in the right direction.

Michael Gnatt learned First Degree Reiki in 1999 and Second Degree in 2005. Although he began integrating Reiki into patient care when he first started practicing, a recent experience with an end-stage cancer patient deepened his appreciation of Reiki's gifts. A patient of his, Karina, had recently been diagnosed with a recurrence of ovarian cancer after being in remission nearly a year. Extensive surgery followed immediately by chemotherapy left her bedridden. Responding to a message from an alarmed neighbor, Gnatt made a house call. He was chagrined to see how weak and distressed Karina was, and recognized there were no medical tools to address the intensity of her suffering. Like Klimenko, Gnatt thought a brief Reiki treatment would at least give his patient momentary relief. He was humbled by the result. Gnatt said,

> This was the first time I experienced that Reiki has its own impact separate from the practitioner. In this situation, there was simply nothing I could do, yet by the end of the treatment, Karina's vitality had improved and she got out of bed. The pain washed away and she came alive again. Afterwards she seemed amazingly well and in good spirits, and gave me a walking tour of her apartment, sharing details of her life in the most charming way.

Klimenko told me of another opportunity she had to use Reiki with a clinic patient, a woman with HIV who came to the clinic after vomiting heavily for several days. The patient had a seizure in the examining room and was very disoriented afterward. Klimenko placed hands on the woman's shoulders to offer Reiki. The patient began sobbing, saying, "I'm sorry, I'm so scared," and refused to be taken to the emergency room (standard medical care after seizures). Although the patient was hysterical, Klimenko knew the change in her patient's self-awareness and ability to communicate was a good sign, and she continued offering Reiki on her back. By the time the ER medics arrived, the woman was smiling. She looked compassionately at one medic and said, "You look so tired." In five minutes of Reiki treatment, the patient had moved from postseizure disorientation through intense emotion to a place of poise that allowed her to be aware of both herself and those around her and to accept the medical help she needed.

COPING WITH CHRONIC ILLNESS

Reiki can be enormously helpful for individuals with chronic, even serious illnesses such as lupus, cystic fibrosis, lymphoma, chronic fatigue syndrome, or Lyme disease. HIV/AIDS provides a striking example, and the way Reiki is used with HIV is relevant to people facing any chronic illness. Many people with HIV/AIDS have long used Reiki to support their well-being and manage the side effects of medications. My first classes training people with HIV/AIDS to practice Reiki were at Gay Men's Health Crisis in New York City in 1994. These classes started before the advent of highly active antiretroviral therapy (HAART), when available medications could address only secondary infections. Besides the fear and constant suffering that HIV/AIDS brought my students, the frequent deaths of friends kept many in a state of continual bereavement. Learning Reiki gave my students a way to relieve their pain and anxiety. (We later documented this benefit—see chapter 13.) It also enabled them to lessen the suffering of the dying. Helping friends meet death peacefully softened the anguish of the survivors' losses.

It was clear that students were benefiting from the Reiki classes, but I wondered what happened after the training ended. A series of follow-up questionnaires I created that were filled out on a voluntary basis showed a trend linking Reiki with improved functioning and decreased pain. The students' tendency was to practice Reiki daily for a while after the class ended, and they reported concurrent reduction of pain and improved functioning. Then, as they got used to feeling better, experiencing less pain and enjoying greater ease of functioning, many slackened their Reiki practice. And guess what happened? Pain increased and functioning took a nosedive. As the students returned to daily Reiki practice, they again reported decreased pain and improved functioning.

REIKI IN EMERGENCY CARE

"It can't hurt. It may help, and that's my job—to help," says Jay Ferrill, paramedic and Second Degree Reiki practitioner. Ferrill is one of an increasing number of medical professionals who use Reiki alongside (never instead of) conventional emergency protocols in ambulances, emergency rooms, and acute-care centers across the country. Reiki's spontaneous, responsive activation enables medics and emergency-room doctors to use Reiki even as their minds are focused on life-and-death medical details.[3] It is often not until a patient is stabilized that first responders who are Reiki trained become aware that Reiki has been active in their hands. Reiki may be invisible, but the results often are not, especially in critical situations.

Nancy Eos, M.D., is a superb example of a physician who has naturally integrated Reiki into patient care. Eos was already a seasoned ER doctor when she learned Reiki in 1990. She began putting her hands on patients more often and watching carefully. A physician who also put herself through law school, Eos wasn't interested in leaps of faith, and she had no vested interest in Reiki's performance, but if Reiki could improve her patients' outcomes, she wanted to know.

Eos approached her experience with Reiki critically, observing carefully to see if her patients benefited, and alert for adverse reactions. Over six years of integrating Reiki into standard emergency care, Eos is convinced that emergency patients who receive even moments of Reiki fare better than those who do not. After offering Reiki, Eos watched patients deviate from the usual medical course. "Their situations improved unexpectedly," Eos says, "following a more gentle course of healing that didn't require procedures as frequently and had less serious outcomes than usual for the same condition." She says, "Patients receiving Reiki almost always improved beyond usual medical expectations."

Of course, this can happen with any individual patient. All physicians in clinical care see some patients recover against enormous odds while others fail unexpectedly. Eos's clinical observation was that Reiki improved her patients' chances of recovery. Realizing the enormity of this observation, Eos followed nearly all the patients she treated with Reiki. She dutifully admitted patients to the departments appropriate to the details in their charts. Once the patients were admitted, however, they often improved so quickly that the physicians assuming their care were unsure why the patients were in the hospital. In a large inner-city hospital, this might never be noticed. But in the small hospital where Eos worked, it was.

Occasionally, Eos placed hands on a patient who had been triaged to low priority and realized he or she was worse off than the nurses thought. At first, the nurses were incredulous when Eos asked for measures not apparently needed, but after watching the outcomes, they came to trust her assessments. Eventually, Eos would hear nurses say, "Nancy, come put your hands on this patient." One case involved a woman who had jumped out of a moving pickup truck, the kind that is elevated on large tires. Although the victim was restless, yelling and screaming, there was scant evidence of injury. When Eos touched the patient to soothe her, her Reiki hands responded so strongly that she had the nurse change the patient's priority status. The increased medical attention uncovered four broken ribs, internal bleeding into the lung, and a cardiac contusion. Reiki seemed to stabilize the patient, and the escalation of medical care saved her life. The patient was sent to the trauma center and released two days later.

Does Eos see any downside to using Reiki in the ER? "There was a time when I went through turmoil trying to figure out how much medicine to use and how much to trust Reiki," she says. "I didn't want to miss giving a medication when I was supposed to, but I also didn't want to overdo the meds. I was constantly contemplating how to walk that line using both Reiki and conventional medicine to come to a better outcome for my patient in an emergency situation."

When a patient arrived in the ER with a level of cardiac distress to warrant TPA, the cardiac medication prescribed to help stop a heart attack, which was at that time $1,000 a shot, Eos would order TPA and offer Reiki while the nurses prepared the medication. By the time a nurse arrived with the injection, the patient no longer required it, she says.

When this happened a second time, Eos realized she needed to offer Reiki *as* she examined these patients.

Physicians have different solutions to the which-to-do-first dilemma they face as medical professionals and Reiki practitioners. Patricia Bailey, M.D., shared hers in the periodical *Hospital Physician*.[4] According to her account, a thirteen-year-old girl who had overdosed on her mother's tricyclic antidepressants arrived in cardiac arrest at the emergency room where Bailey worked. The patient did not have sufficient vital signs to be admitted. Nonetheless, the medical team tried for two hours to resuscitate her. Finally, with no medical options left, Bailey gently placed her hand on the patient's forehead to say good-bye. Bailey was trained in Reiki, and as her hand rested on the girl's forehead, she was surprised to feel Reiki activate. The patient's blood pressure rose sufficiently that she was admitted and taken to cardiac care.

Bailey visited the teen after finishing her ER shift that night. The electroencephalogram was flat, indicating that the patient's brain was not active. It was expected that the girl would be declared legally dead within twenty-four hours. Although Bailey used Reiki at the holistic health clinic where she worked, she did not usually bring Reiki into standard emergency care. Now that she was a visitor rather than a physician, though, she felt she could freely offer Reiki. While receiving Reiki, the patient opened her eyes. She was released a week later. Her only lingering symptom was a minimal cranial nerve palsy.

NOT ONLY THE PATIENTS BENEFIT

Reiki enables clinicians to care for patients in a way that nourishes the caregivers as well, humanizing and even spiritualizing each point of contact. Medical professionals who often have to hurt patients in order to help them are relieved to incorporate Reiki's comforting touch seamlessly into routine care. Reiki quietly includes the care provider in the circle of healing.

Pediatric oncologist John Graham-Pole, M.D., is a professor of pediatrics at the University of Florida in Gainesville and a Reiki practitioner. He finds Reiki to be valuable in palliative care, particularly for children with sickle cell anemia. The experience, he says, is "very rewarding. Offering Reiki allows me to have a very direct connection with the patient in a way that is literally a connection. It's also good for me because it slows me down and gets me to a place where I'm a better healer."

As the relationship with Reiki develops through committed practice over time, practitioners find that the distinction between Reiki pulsations and Reiki consciousness blurs. The practitioner becomes aware of being anchored in that ineffable state, or even catching glimpses of it, at times when Reiki is not being practiced deliberately. Physicians and other professional caregivers find this tremendously supportive, lifting them out of the sea of demands that clinical caregiving can become. They feel supported by a silent partner that encompasses their relationship with the patient rather than pitting them against each other.

Pain specialist James Dillard, M.D., says, "Reiki helps my patients and helps the treatment immensely, but I also feel how much it's helping me. I always have that awareness, which is not inconsequential. Physicians have to stay up to speed for each patient. We can't shlep through our consultations. Reiki feeds the interaction with my patients and keeps me going during the day."

There are so many demands and expectations on physicians and health-care providers. Reiki gives them a way to be with the patient in front of them that, though less results-oriented, ironically, gets better results.

Burnout is a problem in all areas of medicine. The high number of deaths caused by medical error—upward of 44,000 people a year in the United States—suggests we would do well to take better care of our medical personnel. Training them to practice Reiki gives a tool for self-care and a compassionate touch for patient and caregiver alike. Creating a more humane work schedule is complicated, but bringing short Reiki breaks into the workplace need not be.

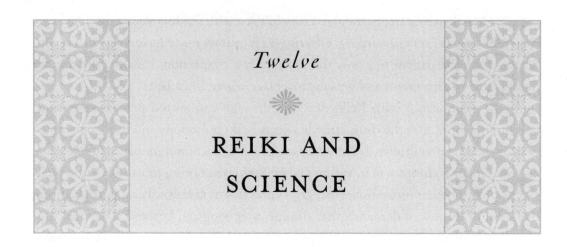

Twelve

REIKI AND SCIENCE

The important thing in science is not so much to obtain new facts
as to discover new ways of thinking about them.

Sir William Bragg

Hawayo Takata, the Reiki master who brought the practice from Japan to America, taught: Remove the cause and there shall be no effect.[1]

Overly simplistic? Unsatisfying? Completely understandable.

The way Reiki works is not as cut-and-dried as many conventional medical treatments, where cause and effect are often clearly defined. To understand how Reiki works, we need to go beyond the scope of conventional medicine—but not beyond the scope of rationality. Rather, we need simply to allow ourselves to extend past the limits of what scientific technology is capable of measuring *at this time*. Considering how dramatically the limits of scientific measurement have changed, this is not magical thinking, nor does it require a leap of faith.

By 1997, nearly half the American population was using complementary and alternative medicine (CAM), and using it a lot: That year, Americans made 629 million visits to CAM practitioners, more visits than they made to primary-care doctors.[2] The National Institutes of Health (NIH) responded to this remarkable statistic by upgrading the Office of Alternative Medicine to the National Center for Complementary and Alternative Medicine (NCCAM), a center devoted to studying these "nonscientific" approaches to healing in order to understand if, when, and how they work, and whether they are safe. In addition, NCCAM makes that research available both to the public and the medical profession, so that effective CAM therapies can be integrated into conventional health care. The government is interested in CAM because it offers not only the promise of greater knowledge of prevention but also safer, less invasive treatments for many medical problems, and such benefits as faster recovery, shorter hospital stays, greater patient and staff satisfaction, and lower costs.

THE TRADITIONAL ROOTS OF MEDICINE

CAM therapies, including Reiki, have grown out of healing traditions. What do I mean by healing traditions? Let me tell you a story. Once upon a time, long before science was even a glint in Descartes' eye, the face of medicine looked very different than it does today. Premodern cultures around the world developed unique indigenous healing traditions, some of which evolved into complex, multitiered systems such as the indigenous medicine of India (Ayurveda), Tibet, and China.

Although the healing traditions of Africa, Native America, and Europe did not gel into coherent regional systems as happened in Asia, they often employed surprisingly advanced techniques, including brain surgery in Africa and acupuncture in America. Ötzi the Iceman was discovered frozen in the Austrian-Italian Alps. He died 5,300 years ago, carrying parasites in his intestines, and medicinal mushrooms in his pouch of a variety known to be effective against those particular parasites.[3]

The Subtle Skills of Healing

Indigenous doctors were trained during long apprenticeships to master healers. Besides learning such things as healing rituals and how to identify and prepare medicines from the natural environment, apprentice healers also learned meditative techniques to hone their intuition, a skill considered essential for effective doctoring.

Physicians practicing medicine before the advent of advanced technology used intuition to observe the complex web of connections underlying material reality—connections that link people to one another, to their environment, and to influences invisible to the human eye.

The Web of Consciousness

It's not as specious as it might sound. These physicians realized that everything, including health and illness, exists within the same vibrational context. This all-embracing vibrational web is held in the subtlest level of reality, which we will call primordial consciousness. Primordial consciousness is immanent in that it can be intuited or experienced directly, but it is also transcendent, in that it is greater than the sum of its manifest parts. Indigenous physicians around the world knew then—and know now—that no healing occurs without accessing this most subtle level of reality, primordial consciousness.

On an individual level, each person interacts directly with primordial consciousness through a subtle vibrational body (sometimes called the etheric or astral body) which science has dubbed the biofield. This biofield surrounds and permeates the physical body. If the biofield becomes disordered, disease and/or other unwanted events occur—nightmares, negative emotions, antisocial behaviors, illnesses, even accidents.

Although it is conceived of differently in different cultures, this subtle vibrational body is recognized in all indigenous medicine. Traditional medicine routinely connects with the biofield during the healing process, for it is here, in luminous consciousness, that both the roots of illness *and* the capacity for personal transformation can be accessed. Whereas scientific medicine looks to reorganize the physical body to cure or manage symptoms—because that's what science can measure—indigenous medicine seeks to also reorganize and refresh the biofield, reaching for the inner roots of outer symptoms and restoring the subtle vibrational balance understood to be the foundation of healing and well-being.

BODY/MIND/SPIRIT AND CONSCIOUSNESS

A maxim in traditional African medicine says it most pithily: There is no healing without a change in consciousness.[4] Without changing consciousness—without creating balance in the vibrational blueprint of manifest reality—people continue to manifest the same physical, mental, emotional, and spiritual imbalances. Consciousness shifts as the connection between the individual's biofield and primordial consciousness is strengthened.

How does a change in consciousness impact a person? The actual event may be dramatic or it may be subtle; but when consciousness shifts toward healing, the change in a person's overall well-being is apparent. The details vary from person to person, of course, but people generally report feeling better about themselves, feeling less alone, seeing life differently, having a greater sense of self-agency. One person may simply feel more love for his wife, another senses possibilities where before there were only obstacles, while a third no longer feels burdened by lingering resentment and is less overwhelmed by life in general. These shifts in consciousness empower people in their healing and, in medical parlance, increase adherence to therapeutic protocols.

Again, this may sound magical at first glance to urban or suburban dwellers who spend their days removed from nature. But even today, people who live close to nature (and many of us who don't) experience a connectedness to it and to one another, a sense of being part of a larger whole that exists on an unseen, yet experiential, level of reality. Those who interact with nature on a daily basis experience it as a pulsing and intensely interconnected living system.

Consciousness is everywhere. It's rather like having music piped throughout your home. In every room you enter, the continuity of the music is waiting for you, and it accompanies you to your next destination. Consciousness is in every room of our lives and every nook and cranny of our minds.

No one in conventional medicine today would deny the power of the mind to affect health (this was not the case a mere twenty years ago). Indigenous, or traditional, medicine explicitly recognizes that our state of mind is affected by our spirit, our aliveness, our vitality, which is in turn affected by our access to primordial consciousness.

Our daily experience with water in all its forms can give us a more concrete understanding of consciousness (water is often used as a metaphor for spirit). Anyone who lives by a body of water knows how refreshing it is to be at water's edge. But we also know what humidity feels like. Just as humidity eventually becomes fog or some other form of precipitation, depending on other unseen influences, the sea of primordial consciousness congeals into our spiritual, mental/emotional, and, finally, physical being. Consciousness in this sense is said to be primordial, nondual, or undifferentiated in that it is singular, the cosmic common denominator. Rather than *being intelligent,* consciousness *is intelligence itself.* Because consciousness is the omnipresent underpinning of manifest reality, what physicists call the unified field, shifts in consciousness are as real as shifts in weather patterns.*

REIKI AND CONSCIOUSNESS

Before we can begin to understand Reiki, we need to understand this use of the word *consciousness,* which is different from the medical use. Of course, one needn't under-

---

*The modern cultural remnants of this belief in nature's aliveness are seen in our sense of the eyes as the windows to the soul. We know how unmistakably health and joy shine through the eyes. Those who work with the dying recognize the stages of death's progress through the loss of luster in the eyes. Indigenous physicians follow this luminosity as it leaves the body, understanding it to be the unchanging continuation of reality, body/mind/spirit, and recognizing that the process of dying isn't complete just because the heart stops.

stand Reiki itself to experience it—and many find the understanding comes more easily after the experience—but a fundamental understanding of the connection between an individual's biofield and primordial consciousness is helpful in contemplating the workings of Reiki.

Primordial consciousness is the source of the healing pulsations we call Reiki. Confusingly for Westerners, the term *Reiki* also refers to primordial consciousness itself, as well as to this particular practice by which Reiki consciousness and Reiki pulsations are accessed. Such ambiguity can be frustrating to Americans, but is very comfortable to the Japanese, whose language is a watercolor of nuance and allusion.

In any case, Reiki can be defined as pure consciousness. It is not restricted to specific pathways in the body. When one applies hands to offer Reiki, consciousness pulsates according to the need of the receiver, like water seeking its own level. As the receiver moves toward balance, Reiki pulsations adjust and eventually become quiet. As a result, the person receiving the treatment moves toward his unique point of balance (as much as is possible at that time).

As pure consciousness, Reiki can be thought of as the embryonic stem cell of subtle vibration (or even energy medicine) in that Reiki appears either to morph into the oscillations that most effectively and gently create balance in the moment, or to become a catalyst precipitating the appropriate cascade of responses needed to balance (experienced practitioners feel varied and changing pulsations as this happens). This is not to imply that Reiki is a panacea, or the only thing that anyone needs at any time. Reiki may, however, always be of benefit in laying the foundation of healing by balancing the biofield and enhancing the connection to primordial consciousness. Although well-being doesn't increase in a strictly linear fashion, Reiki treatment is cumulative, with each session moving the system to greater coherence and integration.

By enhancing our connection to primordial consciousness, Reiki changes our understanding of who we are and what is possible, while increasing our stability and groundedness. As we continue to practice regularly over time, we come to experience ourselves and life itself in a different way. Our appreciation of what is valuable in life changes. This may be reflected in our ambition, enabling us to pursue self-expression at the same time that we value our livelihood for the blessing it is. Many clients of mine have thought that in order to find fulfillment, they needed to change careers; after experiencing Reiki, they realized that they needed only to change their understanding. Reiki practice allowed this transformation in consciousness to unfold gracefully.

"MEASURING" REIKI

Energy medicine is one of the most popular and rapidly growing areas of CAM.[5] Although Reiki is actually more akin to meditation than it is to a medical intervention, and it can be argued that such spiritual practices would be more accurately classified and studied separately, as previously noted, NCCAM has classified Reiki in a subcategory of energy medicine called biofield therapies. Such therapies affect subtle energy fields, which are purported to surround and penetrate the human body.

Because biofields have not yet been measured by reproducible methods, therapies addressing them are referred to as putative. Bioelectromagnetism, sound, light, and other therapies that can be scientifically measured are called veritable. Once scientific measurement of biofield therapies is possible, it may be seen that they are based on the same principles as veritable therapies.*

Meanwhile, why would the government fund the study of biofields, which haven't even been scientifically shown to exist? Good question. It is here that we confront the limitations of science. Don't get me wrong—science is valuable, very valuable, and personally, I love the rigor of scientific inquiry. But science is a tool created by human intelligence; it is not universal law. Not only does science have its limitations, but the unskilled use of science can be very misleading, even damaging.

---

*Researcher and author James Oschman, Ph.D., asserts that biofields have, in fact, been measured. His books *Energy Medicine* and *Energy Medicine in Therapeutics and Human Performance,* are fascinating, in-depth examinations of the field and must-reads for anyone seriously interested in the scientific basis and applications of subtle therapies.

What Can Science Tell Us?

People often think science tells us what is real and what is not. It doesn't. Science measures. It investigates specific questions, called hypotheses, using the scientific method. A hypothesis is a proposition about a relationship between two (or more) things.

Scientific medicine studies interventions such as drugs, herbs, or massage, not to see if they are real—they couldn't be studied if they weren't—but to see if they are beneficial. That is, are they safe and effective? An intervention may be found to be effective but not completely safe, for example. Carefully designed clinical research (research with human subjects) gathers data in the hope of finding at what point the risks of treatment outweigh either the treatment's benefits or the risks associated with the condition or disease. Such measurement guides physicians as they practice medicine.

Yet there are many things that defy measurement. A child's smile, for example. Dreams. As many of you know, a hot flash is real—even if it doesn't show up on a thermometer. Love, too, is real. Many of the best things in life are invisible or immeasurable, but no one doubts they're real.

So the ability to be objectively measured is not a criterion for existence. What is increasingly grabbing the interest of scientists is that things that cannot be measured can indeed affect people in ways that *can* be measured.

The Issue of Measurement

It hasn't been an easy journey to get to this point where science is enlarging its paradigm to include CAM. Given the monopoly science currently has on credibility, it's easy to forget that a mere five centuries ago, scientists themselves were an endangered species chafing under the political power of the Church. Enter René Descartes to the rescue. In the interests of saving science (and scientists), Descartes drew a line in the sand, ostensibly (and as we've come to understand, arbitrarily) dividing reality in two. That which could be measured fell on the side given to science, and that which could not be measured fell on the side given to the Church. Because of this essentially expedient political pronouncement, European thought and culture has been dominated by a belief in the essential dichotomy of science and spirit. The separation of science and spirit strengthened the (misguided) belief in the duality between body and mind that can be traced back to the Greeks.

This mind/body split reached its apogee in the United States, where it seems as embedded in our collective psyche as the separation of Church and state is embedded in our Constitution. It is important to note, however, that only European-based culture imagined this division between body and mind. Everywhere else in the world, including the pre-Columbian native culture of the Americas, the continuity of mind/body/spirit is culturally entrenched and medically utilized.[6]

A lot has changed since the Age of Reason, and time has shown that Descartes knew which side of the line to stand on. Through the grace of—guess what?—scientific technology, the realm of that-which-can-be-measured has increased exponentially. As science extends perception and measurement into increasingly obscure levels of reality—quantum reality and galactic space, for example—it is also slowly eroding belief in the infallibility of measurement and revealing the shortsightedness of ignoring context. In fact, science is coming around to undo the very dichotomy that made it possible for science to survive in the first place. This is happening in three main scientific arenas: in physics (both quantum and theoretical), in frontier science,* and, most surprisingly of all, in biomedicine.

Biomedicine: Science Comes Full Circle

While I am fascinated by quantum physics, superstring theory, and the work of frontier scientists, what really interests me is what is happening in biomedical research. In the last twenty years, there has been much biomedical research conducted in various specialties showing that body/mind/spirit comprise a continuum rather than mutually exclusive categories. (This of course was not what the researchers were targeting.)

---

*Frontier science, as described by the website of the Center for Frontier Sciences at Temple University, uses sound scientific methods to challenge accepted scientific models and perspectives, encouraging "critical review and healthy skepticism."

From a scientific perspective, what is healing but reorganization toward greater coherence? Isn't reorganization that improves a situation itself an indication of intelligence? Reiki, as primordial consciousness, suffuses the receiver with natural intelligence, enhancing its innate ability to reorganize and heal. What is the relationship between the reorganization seen on the physical level and the reorganization that creates balance in the biofield, and a change in consciousness, what a spiritual perspective calls transformation?

By the time I came upon Reiki over twenty years ago, I had enough of a background in traditional, indigenous medical systems and spiritual practice (which are always intertwined) to appreciate the logic behind what was happening to me during a Reiki session. As I practiced Reiki with myself, my family and friends, and my clients, I saw again and again how easily Reiki can make a significant difference in health and well-being. I longed to express this profound, and profoundly simple, spiritual healing practice in biomedical language and to articulate a plausible theoretical model that would help organize existing data, identify gaps in our knowledge, and generate hypotheses to guide needed research.

If we pay attention, it becomes obvious that science is actually pushing the envelope, making us take a more spiritual view of reality, one that takes the unseen and the currently unmeasurable into account. The evidence is in the literature; it's just a matter of gathering it across disciplines and connecting the dots. Science itself is tearing down the false walls between science and spirituality. Nearly 2,500 years ago, Plato said, "Science is nothing but perception." Science is now extending the limits of perception through technology (and nanotechnology) at an unprecedented rate. Data from the new technologies highlight the distortion in our perception. The world is not as it appears, not as plain as the proverbial nose on the face.

VIBRATION

Translating science into common parlance is tricky to begin with; discovering and expressing possible links among different disciplines is even more challenging because each discipline has its own very specialized language, and the language itself can become an obstacle. Often the best we can do is to speak in metaphors to start the conversation, choosing our words carefully and hoping to spark the kind of continued and rigorous dialogue by which both science and collective wisdom are developed. Knowing that so much in our current world was unimaginable a mere half-century ago (for better or worse), we cannot afford to be dismissive of what doesn't fit neatly into the biomedical paradigm. As the nineteenth-century English biologist Thomas Huxley articulated so cogently, "In scientific work, those who refuse to go beyond fact rarely get as far as fact."

Brian Greene, Ph.D., is author of *The Elegant Universe* and *The Fabric of the Cosmos* and star of a three-hour PBS *Nova* special. He is also professor of mathematics and professor of physics at both Columbia and Cornell Universities and codirector of the Institute for Strings, Cosmology and Astroparticle Physics. Greene is as committed to the integrity of his science as he is to conveying the wonders of physics to a broader audience. When I asked him if it would be accurate to say that, according to contemporary physics, vibration is the substratum of reality as we know it, he assured me this was a reasonable statement.

Vibration is an important cornerstone where science and spirituality meet on level ground. Every time you see the word "spiritual," substitute "vibrational" and see if it makes sense. Vibration, or oscillation, is a scientifically sound perspective from which to theorize and research healing, and one that is true to Reiki. *Pulsation* is another word we can use.

These vibrations, pulsations, or oscillations—whatever you want to call them—are the subtle form through which we experience Reiki. They are the *spirit* in spirituality.*

---

*Curiously for two such different languages, the Japanese *rei* nearly equates with *spirit* in English, and has the same ambiguity of referring to ghosts or the most sublime awareness.

MEDICALLY SPEAKING

At this point, you may be asking how, in biomedical terms, does Reiki work? We don't yet know. However, scattered among various medical specialties, I have come upon biomedical research data relevant to this topic, data that make the chemical-mechanistic model seem inadequate to explain the plasticity and complexity of the human body and that make a holistic model—complete with underlying conditions and split-second systemic communication—seem more plausible.

Regenerative Medicine

Science has come a long way in demonstrating the plasticity of the human system since researchers at the Pasteur Institute in Paris in the 1920s first showed that the immune system responds to classical Pavlovian conditioning. We now know that actions and experiences shape the brain and influence gene expression.

But science has yet to discover how/why embryonic stem cells "know" to differentiate into the complexity of the human (or animal) body or why a predictable process of cellular scattering and reorganization occurs in cell repair.[7] Nonetheless, regenerative medicine is looking to capitalize on this intelligence. There is now evidence that not only the cells of bone marrow, liver, kidney, and nerves regenerate, but also the heart and the insulin-producing cells of the pancreas. However, researchers working independently of one another have documented the unwillingness of healthy cells to regenerate into a damaged or diseased area. The Miami Project to Cure Paralysis at the University of Miami School of Medicine, under the direction of Mary Bunge, Ph.D., is trying to coax nerve cells to regenerate across the site of injury, while Piero Anversa, M.D., a researcher at New York Medical College, faces a similar dilemma in the human heart. According to Anversa, there is continuous regeneration of cells in the heart that is potentiated when there is a problem (primitive heart cells can be found regenerating next to the damaged area of the heart up to twenty-four hours after death). Like nerve cells, however, the regenerating heart cells don't move into the area of injury on their own.[8]

Robert O. Becker, M.D., author of *The Body Electric* and *Cross Currents,* and twice nominated for a Nobel Prize, was a pioneer of bioelectromagnetism, the study of how electromagnetic fields interact with life. Becker compared the healing of salamanders, which regenerate, with that of frogs, which while just one step higher on the evolutionary scale, have lost the ability to regenerate. The electrical current at the threshold of regeneration is negative. Frogs, which like humans simply seal the amputation site, generate a positive current. Although much was left unknown, Becker's continuing experiments unmasked electromagnetic energy as a controlling factor in healing. Might bioelectromagnetism be implicated in the failure of nerve and heart cells to move into the damaged site?

Meanwhile, in the immunobiology lab at Massachusetts General Hospital, director Denise Faustmann, M.D., ran into a similar obstacle when transplanting insulin-producing islet cells into naturally diabetic mice. Her solution included training the immune-system cells in the blood not to attack islet cells.

Holism sees a corollary to the unwillingness of healthy cells to migrate into an unhealthy area: the possibility of creating the body as a healthy environment in which diseased cells cannot flourish.

Cell Communication

On another front, Guenter Albrecht-Buehler, Ph.D., of Northwestern University Medical School, has studied cell intelligence for more than two decades. His research has revealed that cells read their environment through signals of near-infrared light and adjust accordingly. According to Albrecht-Buehler, near infrared light seems to be the physical carrier of a "language" that is nonphysical, which may be a modulation or pulsing of the light. He suggests that in the future, it might be possible to use the cells' language to direct them to migrate across a damaged area.

According to researcher James L. Oschman, Ph.D., the crystalline lattice of the connective tissue (fascia) emits bioelectronic signals unique to the tissue and to the particular way in which it is being moved or manipulated. The connective tissue is a semiconducting communication network that runs throughout the body. In addition,

Oschman told me, "The body is a gigantic water antenna."[9] The body continually receives and processes signals both from the environment and from its own movement. This opens a scientific basis for understanding a range of subtle therapies such as homeopathy, aromatherapy, and Reiki, and even the practice of yoga postures.

Is there a common denominator among these data? The scientific community is so fragmented into areas of specialty that it is often unable to connect the dots between such studies and make broad use of what has been learned. And research has yet to focus on the mechanisms and process of healing. Without a paradigm of health or an institute of healing, we have only isolated bits of knowledge, sometimes orphaned as anomalous data. Einstein pointed out, "It is theory that decides what can be observed." The first step is to articulate a plausible theoretical model with which to organize existing data that is anomalous in a paradigm of disease but meaningful in a model of health.

A HOLISTIC MODEL OF HEALTH

Asian medicine has such a model, one that is in some ways an extended version of the biomedical model and which holds the complexity and plasticity of the human system. Unlike the biomedical model, the holistic model anticipates breakthroughs. That means that we don't have to throw out what we used to "know" every time new data arrive. Asian medicine has developed clinical practices based on theoretical models that include no uncaused phenomena and that describe the processes of maintaining and of regaining health. Meanwhile, biomedical science is trying to prove Asian medicine on biomedicine's terms. This will bring limited success because the holistic paradigm of traditional medicine, with its focus on overall well-being and optimal functioning, is larger than the paradigm of biomedicine, with its more limited focus on disease and injury.

Although we do not yet know the mechanism of action for Reiki, there are promising avenues for research to explore. It appears that Reiki interacts with the body's control center, whatever is understood to fulfill that function, thereby enhancing the body's self-regulatory mechanisms and innate healing ability. Whereas pharmaceuticals tend to impose a unidirectional effect on the body, Reiki acts as a vibrational adaptogen, an agent that encourages the individual system to balance regardless of the skew of the imbalance. Functioning that is sluggish gets stimulated, that which is erratic becomes stable, and that which is high-strung is soothed. Flaxseed is an example of adaptogenic food. It moves the bowels of someone who is constipated, but it also relieves diarrhea. The mechanism through which flaxseed works is well known, but that of adaptogenic herbs such as ginseng and rhodiola rosea has scientists befuddled. Andrew Weil, M.D., suggests that perhaps such tonic herbs offer the body a wide range of nutrients from which it intelligently chooses what is needed. Given that the workings of even adaptogenic herbs that can be analyzed in the laboratory remain a mystery, it is not surprising that science does not yet understand the adaptogenic effect of Reiki.

Reiki has a near-immediate impact on nervous-system functioning. Traditional Asian medicine appreciates that impacting the nervous system has broad implications for health, and conventional medicine agrees. Maybe this will help explain why Reiki benefits people irrespective of their symptomatology and their awareness. Existing research, while limited, shows promising effects of Reiki on anxiety and pain, two conditions that biomedicine links with the nervous system.

GUT INTELLIGENCE

Biomedicine has long had knowledge of the gut that does not neatly fit the biomedical model and which has subsequently been largely ignored. The gut has a nervous system of its own, called the enteric nervous system, that interacts directly with the immune system without requiring input from the brain or the spinal cord. The enteric nervous system communicates with the brain through the tenth cranial nerve, called the vagus nerve. The vagus nerve mediates the parasympathetic nervous system, which heals and recharges the body. Epilepsy and depression can be treated by vagus nerve stimulation, which can also improve learning and memory.

Michael Gershon, M.D., professor and chair of the department of anatomy and cell biology at Columbia University College of Physicians and Surgeons, is a noted researcher of the enteric nervous system. According to him, "The gut itself contains more nerve cells than exist in the rest of the peripheral nervous system." In addition, "the gut has been shown to be able to work independently even if all nerves to it are cut; there is reflex activity in a test tube." Gershon refers to the enteric nervous system as the second brain, not because it thinks cognitively, but rather because it affects the functioning of the brain. Furthermore, he says, the gut (the entire bowel, from mouth to anus) is the largest immune organ of the body.

This information about the enteric nervous system dovetailed with my clinical experience and with the perspective of Asian medical systems. In years of practicing Reiki, I've seen various gut pathologies such as irritable bowel syndrome and Crohn's disease respond beautifully to treatment. This made sense from the traditional perspective, in which the physical nervous system and its subtle component are implicated in any imbalanced state and are linked to the large intestine. (In traditional medicine, health and disease always involve both the physical body and nonphysical rest of us, so there is none of the dismissiveness conventional medicine has historically attached to the psychosomatic.) The entire nervous system is a place where the traditional model and the biomedical model converge. It is of further interest because, as Gershon says, when it comes to irritable bowel syndrome, "most conventional forms of treatment have one thing in common, failure."

ENHANCING SYSTEMIC FLOW

A holistic perspective sees health as a resilient and dynamic state characterized by balanced flow throughout the biofield. Irregularities in biofield circulation—either too fast or too sluggish—correspond with declining health. This connection between balanced flow and health is also seen in the biomedical model. Reiki seems to improve flow on many levels. For example, the breath slows and deepens within minutes of starting Reiki treatment and nurses remark on how patients receiving Reiki "pink up."

When a system as complex as a human being responds as quickly as it does to Reiki, it's likely that science will uncover multiple avenues of action requiring a systems research approach. The speed and nonlocality of response suggest the possibility of entrainment or resonance involving the vagus nerve; the chemical-mechanistic model is too slow to account for such responsiveness.

What is happening biochemically and quantumly during these experiences? Researchers are beginning to explore the biochemical responses to Reiki treatment, which are discussed in chapter 13. We don't know what's happening at the quantum level, nor is it likely that Reiki will show up on the radar of research physicists any time soon. In the meantime, it is reasonable to theorize that as part of the mechanism of balancing the individual and increasing coherence—removing the cause to remove the effect—Reiki might be involved in the alignment of quantum events. Enhancing order in the quantum underpinning of material reality might lead to what physicists call a "phase change," a minuscule adjustment that tips the scale to a discernible change such as happens when water freezes to ice. This is pure hypothesis to create a conceptual bridge where we lack data. It is, however, plausible and fits both the quantum and the biomedical models. As such it is a hypothesis worth investigating.

Does the sense of well-being that accompanies the relaxation of a typical Reiki treatment influence the functioning of the immune system, which is well documented to be affected by emotional states? Are we seeing a simple normalization process, precipitating a cascade of events by which overall functioning is balanced? And if so, how is that evidenced at a molecular level?

Since Reiki is vibration, is it a subtle form of sound or a precursor of sound? According to texts of nondualist philosophy,[10] consciousness emerges as vibration that displays the qualities of light and sound, but that is not seen as separate from pure consciousness (Reiki is traditionally understood to be both the pulsations and the source of the pulsations). Might Reiki be an inaudible hum, akin to the sound of OM, which yogis call the primordial sound of the universe? Might the benefits of Reiki be related to the healing effects of chanting and drones such as the didgeridoo of the Australian aborigine or the tamboura of classical Indian music? The cross-cultural prevalence of toning in healing and spiritual practices is hard to discount, and it is supported by data from a range of studies. For example, a UCLA study found that hospitalized schizophrenics who hummed *"mmmm"* had a 60 percent reduction in auditory hallucinations.[11] Humming creates sound waves that reverberate throughout the sinuses like a subtle inner massage, helping to clear secretions and promote air flow.[12] Humming seems to stimulate the production of nitric oxide, which helps stimulate immune response and regulate blood pressure, and affects communication among brain neurons. Nitric-oxide levels in the sinuses of healthy participants were fifteen times greater when they hummed rather than when they breathed without making noise.[13] Additionally, the benefits of ultrasound are well documented.* Clearly vibration has widespread application to healing.

WHAT A HOLISTIC BIOMEDICAL MODEL COULD PROVIDE

Creating a model relevant to both biomedicine and traditional healing requires collaboration of scientists and practitioners of different backgrounds and philosophies. The model underlying traditional medical systems is both plausible and somewhat similar to the biomedical model. Since the holistic model extends beyond that which can be measured scientifically to include subtler levels of reality, it offers the ability to detect imbalance before it becomes embedded in the body as pathology, and restore balance. This opens the possibility not only of less invasive therapeutic procedures but also of effective prevention.

---

*According to Chukuka Enwemeka, Ph.D., dean of the School of Health Professions, Behavioral and Life Sciences at New York Institute of Technology, the cellular response to light and sound enhances healing at a certain interval in the healing process. At the time when cells are dividing and producing collagen, they respond to ultrasound by dividing faster and producing collagen faster. Enwemeka says it appears that the cells somehow access the sound energy to enhance the energy available to them to make this effort. Light and sound are two distinct forms of energy. They both vibrate, but they vibrate in different ways.

The increased awareness of underlying conditions and the intelligent interconnectedness of the human system point toward a holistic model and support Takata's explanation, remove the cause and you will eliminate the effect. Traditional medical systems explain pathogenesis in great detail. Resulting treatment is highly individualized and multilayered.

Conventional biomedicine can take a simple step toward incorporating the broader view of traditional medical systems by taking advantage of the overall balancing effect of Reiki, which addresses not only a person's underlying health imbalance but also the unbalancing side effects of conventional pharmacology and procedures. Even when surgery is a lifesaving necessity, it still delivers a profound shock to the system, one that puts the patient at greater risk of dying *of apparently unrelated causes* in the year or two after surgery.[14] Reiki can extend the reach of biomedicine without getting in the way.

Physicist Brian Greene says, "Our deepest intuitive awareness of truth that guides science at its best knows it is not possible that there is one set of laws for galactic universe (theory of relativity) and another for subatomic reality (quantum theory). This is why we reach for a unifying theory that postulates over-arching law, one master principle that could govern everything."

A unifying theory of everything will include not only galactic and subatomic space, it will also include biomedicine. This will not undo all that biomedicine knows; it will enhance that body of knowledge and explain much data that is homeless in the current, limited paradigm.

Thirteen

REIKI AND
MEDICAL RESEARCH

*Not everything that counts can be counted, and not
everything that can be counted counts.*

ALBERT EINSTEIN

A Chinese maxim advises, "For those who don't believe, there is never enough proof, and for those who believe, no proof is necessary." Between those extremes lie a number of inquisitive, caring, and truly open-minded physicians who wait for research results that are slow to arrive.

As physicians begin to grasp the paradigm of holistic medicine, they can develop a sense of what is likely to be safe and where more caution is needed, as well as how to recognize skilled healers with whom they might collaborate and how to identify the sometimes subtle benchmarks of healing. They still need hard evidence that Reiki improves clinical outcomes and is cost-effective. Any treatment not shown to be effective from a scientific perspective is much less likely to be offered to patients or to be reimbursed by medical insurance policies. So there are very practical reasons why it is important to research the effects of Reiki.

There is also the larger picture. As Andrew Weil, M.D., points out, "Any research that shows a nonphysical approach can change a physical system is extremely significant in that it challenges the predominant paradigm that says only a physical intervention can produce a physical change in the system. I would like to see medicine become less committed to that materialistic viewpoint, and research in energy medicine is one of the ways in which that can happen."[1]

While research on Reiki is clearly valuable, the research tools developed to investigate pharmaceuticals are not necessarily appropriate to the study of holistic therapies, for many complex reasons. Spearheaded often by physicians who have seen patients benefit from CAM therapies, researchers are looking for ways to address the challenges traditional healing therapies present to conventional research models.[2] While it may be true that the most profound benefits Reiki offers are simply not measurable, there are aspects of Reiki treatment that can and should be studied. Let's look first at what has been done, and then discuss what other research might be done.

As with most complementary therapies, research on Reiki is in its infancy. The literature so far consists of case reports, descriptive studies, and randomized control trials (RCTs) done with a small number of patients.* As of this writing, no large RCTs studying the clinical effects of Reiki have been published.[3] The NIH's National Center for Complementary and Alternative Medicine has to date five studies looking at Reiki's effectiveness in reducing stress and helping patients with advanced AIDS, diabetes, fibromyalgia, and prostate cancer.[4]

Responses to Reiki treatment can be measured both objectively and through self-report (used to measure, for example, pain, quality of life, and satisfaction with treat-

---

*Reiki—Review of a Biofield Therapy: History, Theory, Practice and Research" is a medical review of Reiki I cowrote with Gala True, Ph.D., senior researcher at Albert Einstein Healthcare Network in Philadelphia, which was published in the peer-reviewed medical journal *Alternative Therapies in Health & Medicine* 9, no. 2 (March/April 2003): 62–72, and which provides a more in-depth look at the research up to that date.

ment). To date, there have been some interesting smaller studies that, while far from conclusive, have had promising results.

In general, studies have found Reiki to be associated with:

- decreased levels of stress hormones
- improvement in immune indicators
- improved blood pressure
- subjective improvements in anxiety, pain, and fatigue
- decreased heart rate
- improvement in mood and functioning of depressed patients
- overall enhanced well-being and increased vitality

These effects have been shown whether Reiki is given in person or at a distance, and the effects are not seen in participants receiving sham-Reiki. Among the many populations that are thought to benefit from Reiki are some of those whom medical science considers hardest to treat—those with fibromyalgia and AIDS, and victims of heart attacks. The benefits of Reiki can—and are—being delivered in the most stressful of settings—the cardiac-care unit, the delivery room, the operating room, intensive-care units, and the emergency room.

EXAMPLES OF PROMISING REIKI STUDIES

Biological Indications of Relaxation and Immune Strength

In a study of twenty-three healthy people receiving a thirty-minute Reiki treatment that was published in *Alternative Therapies in Health and Medicine* in 2001, researchers Wardell and Engebretson found significant healthful changes in biological indications of relaxation (actual physiologic and biochemical changes that occur when we relax

and that profoundly affect health) and immune response. During the study, the participants' anxiety and systolic blood pressure dropped significantly (meaning the change
was strong enough that it was unlikely to be caused by chance—an indicator of a valid
finding). There was also a significant improvement in immune response as measured
by increased salivary IgA, the antibody secreted in saliva that protects against infection.

Another interesting finding in this study was a small, not statistically significant,
decrease in blood levels of cortisol. Cortisol is a hormone that the body produces in response to stress, and consistently high levels are known to be unhealthy. For example,
elevated cortisol in breast cancer survivors has been linked to decreased longevity.
Any therapy that shows a trend toward lowered cortisol levels is worth noting, and
further research is warranted.[5]

A randomized study of forty-five participants found the Reiki group had a significant decrease in heart rate and diastolic blood pressure compared to both the control
and the placebo (sham Reiki) group.[6] In another study on cancer patients, Reiki treatment reduced heart rate and diastolic blood pressure.[7]

Improved Management of Cancer Symptoms

Cancer patients frequently suffer from fatigue, pain, and anxiety.[8] A study comparing
Reiki to rest found patients receiving Reiki treatment had significantly reduced fatigue, pain and anxiety, and improved quality of life compared to those who rested.[9]
A study looking at Reiki compared to rest to support standard opioid treatment for
cancer patients at end of life found reduced pain on the days Reiki treatment was
given, and improved quality of life overall for the Reiki group (cited earlier in chapter;
see note 7).

Reduced Pain and Anxiety

Women having hysterectomies who received three thirty-minute Reiki treatments
(one before and two after surgery) asked for less pain medication and reported less

pain after surgery, and less anxiety when leaving the hosptial three days later than women who did not receive Reiki.[10]

A program evaluation of my hospital HIV classes showed Reiki can help manage pain and anxiety. Outpatients were referred to Reiki classes by their primary-care physicians or psychiatrists as support for drug detox and to help manage insomnia, anxiety, and pain. Visual Analog Scale and State-Trait Anxiety Inventory[11] questionnaires filled out by thirty students before and immediately after twenty-minute Reiki treatments showed a significant reduction in pain and anxiety whether students practiced self-treatment or received treatment from another student.[12]

Wardell and Engebretson collected subjective data as well as the objective data noted above. Participants receiving Reiki reported a sense of inner calm, and heightened awareness, and a feeling of having bonded with the Reiki practitioner. This is of note because the treatments were given in a setting similar to those of standard healthcare visits, that is, the participants received treatment from a practitioner they had just met, the sessions were only thirty minutes long, and they were interrupted by the biological measurements being taken. That the objective measures of the Reiki treatment held up in a hospital setting that was not conducive to relaxation is important.[13]

The researchers noted what they called the paradoxical nature of the Reiki experience, for example, feelings of deep relaxation *and* a heightened sense of awareness. Some participants also reported feeling that they were hovering between sleep and awareness during the Reiki treatments. The researchers identified this as a "liminal" state of consciousness and astutely noted such an experience is commonly linked to spiritual states and healing rituals from a wide range of cultures. They proposed that the subjectivity of the experience, while difficult to study empirically, may be critical to its effectiveness.

Depression

The effectiveness of Reiki treatment to support people experiencing various types of depression was the focus of Adina Goldman Shore's doctoral research, published in the journal *Alternative Therapies in Health and Medicine*.[14] Forty-six participants were randomly assigned to one of three treatment groups: hands-on Reiki, distance (Second Degree, nontouch) Reiki, and distance placebo Reiki. The three groups were assessed before and after treatment with standardized psychological assessments (Beck Depression Inventory, Beck Hopelessness Scale, and Perceived Stress Scale).

Participants receiving weekly Reiki treatment for six weeks reported significant reduction in depression, hopelessness, and self-perceived stress, compared with the placebo group. There was no significant difference between the groups receiving Reiki; both the hands-on and the distant Reiki treatment groups improved to a similar degree compared with the placebo group. Perhaps most important, the benefit held when the participants were retested a year later even though they had received no further treatment. In light of the strong result, it is important to note that the researcher characterized all participants as being "highly motivated to participate in their own healing process."

Research Done in Hospital by Staff Care Providers

Reiki practitioners who are part of academic medical centers are in a position to increase the volume and quality of clinical research studies. The following are two small, as yet unpublished, studies that were approved by their respective institutional review boards (IRBs) and implemented in the hospital.

Cheri Herrmann, an RN at New York Hospital Queens (NYHQ), gave brief Reiki treatment to twenty pregnant women admitted to the hospital with either early labor or preeclampsia who also were given standard medical care, magnesium sulfate intravenous therapy (Epsom salts). Women receiving this therapy often complain of side effects such as headache, visual disturbances, and lethargy. Reiki treatment was associated with a significant reduction in the following categories of symptoms: feeling emotionally drained, feeling physically tense, headache, exhaustion, and visual discomfort (eye pain, eye pressure, blurred vision). Reiki is now recognized as an effective intervention for stress management at NYHQ and a Reiki program has started in the labor unit.

There is strong evidence that stress increases risk of cardiac arrhythmia. A healthy heart doesn't beat like a mechanical drum; it has a natural variability in its rhythm, called heart rate variability (HRV). Flattening of HRV in patients who have suffered a heart attack is a strong predictor of poor medical outcomes, even stronger than an elevated heart rate.

Yale medical student Rachel Friedman studied the effect of Reiki on patients who had had heart attacks within the previous seventy-two hours. Forty-eight patients in the cardiac ICU or the cardiac step-down unit were randomized to receive either twenty minutes of Reiki or one of two control treatments. Reiki treatment significantly improved HRV and self-reported anxiety when compared to both control groups and to each subject's own baseline levels. Friedman says, "I'm very excited about the implications this study holds for future research. Reiki appears to be both feasible and effective in a real-life clinical setting."

REIKI AND MASSAGE RELIEVE CANCER-RELATED DISTRESS

Reiki may not be identified as such in all studies, or Reiki may be combined with gentle massage or other therapies. A large study (1,290 patients) published in the *Journal of Pain and Symptom Management* by Barrie R. Cassileth , Ph.D., and Andrew J. Vickers, Ph.D., of Memorial Sloan-Kettering Cancer Center (MSKCC) in New York City documented the effectiveness of touch therapies to control symptoms for inpatients and outpatients. (All massage therapists at MSKCC are also Reiki-trained.) Three types of massage were used: Swedish, light touch, and foot massage. Light touch includes Reiki. Inpatients received twenty-minute treatment, and outpatient treatments were sixty minutes long. Anxiety, fatigue, and pain were most commonly reported as the strongest symptom, in that order. Even patients who gave high scores to their symptoms experienced that the intensity of symptoms after treatment was half what it had been. The authors note that the benefits are likely underrated, since not all patients complained of high levels of all symptoms. The strongest benefit was found for anxiety, but even the weakest benefit, for fatigue, was significant at 43 percent. There was some increase after the initial drop, but the intensity of symptoms did not return to what it had been during the forty-eight-hour period in which participants were monitored.[15]

(NOT) FOR PRACTITIONERS ONLY

The following section is particularly relevant for those interested in research, especially advanced Reiki practitioners and other health-care professionals who may actually be involved in researching Reiki.

WHAT RESEARCH DO WE NEED, AND WHO CAN DO IT?

While documenting the biological changes that occur during Reiki treatment in healthy people and in those with specific medical conditions, it's important for researchers to keep in mind that Reiki does not address disease; Reiki encourages the person toward balance. Given the strength of the anecdotal evidence and Reiki's widespread use in hospitals and by the public, it seems pragmatic to leave aside the question of mechanism of action for the moment and focus on Reiki's effectiveness. Research teams should consist of at least three professionals: a medical professional, a researcher, and an experienced Reiki practitioner. Let's look at some areas worth investigating.

Can Reiki Facilitate the Delivery of Conventional Health Care?

Medical treatment plans and medications are helpful only if the patient actually follows them, and adherence is not as high as physicians would like. Can Reiki help?

How might a few minutes of Reiki affect the experience of health-care visits for patients? Reiki could be offered to patients as they wait for their health-care appointment.

All patients and health-care professionals would rate various aspects of the visits, such as satisfaction with the interaction, on a simple visual analog scale (VAS) immediately after the appointment ends. Patients who did not receive Reiki and the staff who cared for them would fill out the same questionnaires, and the two sets would be compared.

Self-efficacy, the feeling that we can make decisions and take actions that make a difference in our lives, is linked to improved outcomes for patients in need of changing a wide range of behaviors. If Reiki self-treatment were shown to have an effect on self-efficacy, it would be a strong argument to include Reiki in treatment for a range of conditions, including smoking cessation, recovery from addictions, and weight loss.

How does teaching patients Reiki self-treatment affect their medical care and their overall health? Does it engage them in self-care and improve medical outcomes? Does Reiki increase adherence, helping patients complete treatment protocols and courses of medication? Does training adults, teens, and children with chronic illness such as asthma to practice Reiki self-treatment build stability and resilience as they practice regularly over time? Might it also lessen reliance on medications?

Further data is needed from large studies of the effectiveness of Reiki treatment to reduce stress. Such data should include biological effects of treatment along the lines of the Wardell and Engebretson and the Scottish studies.

Can Reiki Affect Medical Outcomes?

The use of Reiki in crisis medicine—ER, OR, ICU, and NICU—is documented in medical literature. These are logical settings for clinical studies, since the more acute the situation, the more likely it is that the response to Reiki will be measurable.

Surgery is an obvious place to document the benefits Reiki can bring patients. Some parameters to study are length of hospital stay, amount of pain medication, and rate of organ rejection, which would be compared with the same variables in control subjects.

Observational studies of birth statistics (length of delivery and hospital stay, medication, maternal satisfaction) of women using Reiki during pregnancy and birth and how they compare with appropriate controls could show that Reiki can provide relief for women in labor. Who better to administer Reiki than the very nurses, doctors, and midwives whom women already trust for their care, especially since Reiki can be offered simultaneously with conventional care?

Can Reiki Help Manage Chronic Illness?

Medical patients with Crohn's disease or diabetes might be studied to see whether they experience not only symptomatic improvement, but also fewer complications and relapses. Does Reiki simply relieve the acute pain of sickle-cell anemia, or do children report fewer pain episodes when they practice Reiki self-treatment regularly?

When researching Reiki's applicability to patients with chronic illness, consider teaching the patients First Degree Reiki. Empowering people who have chronic illness with a skill they can use to manage symptoms and reduce stress has far-reaching benefits and is most cost-effective. By improving well-being, consistent Reiki self-treatment might also lead to behavioral changes that could improve medical outcomes.

Can Reiki Improve Employee Attendance?

Health-care businesses (and others) might be interested to train staff and compare absences in the year before and after using Reiki. Studying the effects of self-treatment avoids any confounding effects of the practitioner-patient relationship.

RESEARCH CONSIDERATIONS SPECIFIC TO REIKI

The lack of standardized training needs to be addressed when researchers study Reiki. Without standardized training, there is no way to compare one practitioner with another. Even if training is standardized, a Reiki master is not necessarily a stronger or "better" practitioner. In addition, Reiki activates according to the need of the individual receiving treatment. For these reasons, I suggest studying Reiki at the First Degree level. Either Reiki works or it doesn't; we don't need Reiki masters or even Second Degree practitioners to get results. The closest we can get to uniformity among practitioners is to train the practitioners as part of the research project. If health-care professionals are trained, they already have the clinical experience needed to work with patients. If patients or healthy people who are not health-care professionals are trained, the effect of self-treatment could be studied.

IN VITRO RESEARCH

I had an opportunity to make an exploratory incursion into a respected laboratory. My student and I held in our hands a series of petri dishes containing cells in various environments in standard use in labs. I requested that a set of dishes containing cells in a non-nourishing environment be included. The cells in the non-nourishing environment responded more than those in any of the nourishing environments. It seems reasonable that the non-nourished cells were in greatest stress, so their response was in keeping with clinical experience that the more dire the circumstances, the more dramatic the response to Reiki.

Although studying the effect of Reiki in vitro may be tempting, I doubt that it is the best way to demonstrate Reiki's effectiveness. Petri dishes don't represent the complexity of a living human, animal, or plant environment. One of Reiki's greatest clinical advantages is that it is a simple practice that can influence complex systems toward balance. What is the system in a petri dish?

RESEARCH FUNDING

Does Reiki affect the production of dopamine, a brain chemical essential to central nervous system functioning? What about endorphins and enkephalins, natural substances involved in the body's own pain control mechanisms? Does Reiki influence the expression of DNA? I would love to know these answers, but who will do the research, and who will fund it?

Nearly $95 billion is spent on medical research in the United States each year, more than what is spent in any other country. Fifty-seven percent of that money comes from drug companies and 28 percent from the NIH.[16] With pharmaceuticals, the burden of research is on the drug companies (and we won't go into the many issues that come up when research is sponsored by business with a vested interest in the results). But who has a profit incentive to research Reiki? Funding comes only from the government, from NCCAM, and grants are very competitive.

Since Reiki treatment is inexpensive compared with pharmaceuticals and medical procedures, much valuable research could be done on a relatively low budget, but practitioners without an academic affiliation have little chance of receiving funding. If Reiki were shown to reduce treatment costs, insurance companies would gain by reimbursing patients for Reiki treatment, at least in specific situations.

IMPROVING RESEARCH COLLABORATION

Since academic medicine is just beginning to recognize the value of CAM, the most experienced CAM practitioners rarely have academic credentials. To create viable, accurate research, bridges need to be built. CAM practitioners interested in research need to educate themselves about the scientific method. We also need access to medical libraries, which are now available only to academics. Medical researchers need to learn how to recognize expertise that lies outside the scope of academic credentials. Outreach to experienced, credible CAM practitioners is crucial to creating credible, rigorous, and meaningful research. These practitioners need to be involved in every stage of research design, execution, and interpretation, and compensated as consultants. Academic researchers are on staff; CAM practitioners are more likely in private practice. The time they spend in collaboration with academics is uncompensated, reducing incomes that are already below those of academics. CAM practitioners need to be paid. We won't have true integrative medicine until we integrate the money.

Effective outreach would identify grassroots research opportunities and empower potential researchers with basic science mentoring and access to statisticians. Basic grassroots documentation could prove valuable in choosing treatments and conditions to study more rigorously.

Under the direction of Jeffrey D. White, M.D., the Office of Cancer Complementary and Alternative Medicine (OCCAM) of the National Cancer Institute of the National Institutes of Health is making promising headway in improving the quality of CAM research. I have been invited to participate in two of their programs. The first was a focus group held during the First International Conference of the Society for Integrative Oncology in New York City in November 2004. A diverse group of medical and CAM practitioners shared their perspectives and frustrations honestly and respectfully. All agreed on the need for rigorous research that reflects a deep understanding of the therapies being studied.

More recently, I was invited to present at OCCAM's October 2007 conference, Cancer Researchers and CAM Practitioners: Fostering Collaborations; Advancing the Science. This two-day conference identified the challenges to high-quality research, offered examples of how these challenges are being met, and gave NCI staff, medical clinicians/researchers, and CAM practitioners an opportunity to present their work and create working relationships. Videocast conference sessions can be viewed at www.cancer.gov/CAM/news/conference2007.html.

Sponsoring such exploratory conversation among professionals of various relevant fields is necessary to improving the quality of research, making it more relevant to the clinical practice of both standard medical treatment and traditional healing therapies, and to the needs of patients. OCCAM is pioneering a pragmatic course through the tangle of CAM research and patients' needs that can be a beacon for other agencies.

RESEARCH YOU CAN DO
WITH YOUR CLIENTS

Reiki practitioners who want to contribute to the knowledge base can do so with a little preparation and minimal expense. Prepare questionnaires for your clients to fill out before and after treatment. Create a form with simple demographic categories, such as age, sex, ethnicity, educational level, and the condition or situation that occasions Reiki. You can create your own questionnaire if you like, but results are more valuable if standard scales are used when available. You may want to include a visual analog scale (VAS) to record changes in pain, and an anxiety scale to measure changes in the client's level of anxiety, as I used in the HIV study. You could use a VAS to measure the effectiveness of the session in improving the condition or situation that brought the client to you.

VAS

What is your pain RIGHT NOW?

No Pain -- Worst Possible Pain
0   1   2   3   4   5   6   7   8   9   10

Data collected by the practitioner are not considered reliable, so arrange a post office box or third-party location where questionnaires can be mailed. Decide if you want to collect data before and immediately after the session only, or if you want to collect a third set of data a few days later. Prepare the questionnaires in advance. If you are collecting three sets of data, include a space for the client to specify how long it has been since the Reiki treatment. Specify an area for additional comments if desired.

Mark two or three identical sets with the same client number so that the before and after responses can be compared, and provide stamped, addressed envelopes for each set. To protect the client's anonymity, don't record the client number. The cleanest, most respectable data are gathered when the client knows responses are anonymous. Unless the client is confident that the questionnaires are anonymous, the responses might be skewed by a desire to please the practitioner.

Before you start the session, give the client a few minutes to fill out the first set of questionnaires and seal it in the envelope. It's important that the client seal the pre-session responses and not reread them before marking the post-session responses.

In order to protect against bias and to keep a fair sample, ask all your new clients at their first visit only. Explain that the purpose of the study is to increase knowledge of Reiki's effectiveness. Be clear that participation is optional and anonymous, and that it will not affect your relationship if the patient chooses not to participate. If you don't ask because you feel the client wouldn't give good responses, the point of the study is undermined.

CONCLUSION

While we are chewing on research possibilities, with the accent on possibility, people are suffering. What more do we need to know before we offer patients Reiki?* On the basis of strong anecdotal evidence, scant research data, and a lack of medical con-

---

*The following are other papers in the medical literature that can help educate physicians and health-care clinicians and administrators about the use of Reiki in conventional health-care settings: Pamela Miles, "Palliative Care Service at the NIH Includes Reiki and Other Mind-Body Modalities," *Advances in Mind Body Medicine* 20, no. 2 (Summer 2004): 3. "Pamela Miles: Reiki Vibrational Healing," Interview by Bonnie Horrigan, *Alternative Therapies in Health and Medicine* 9, no. 4 (July/August 2003): 74–83. Robert Schiller, "Reiki: A Starting Point for Integrative Medicine," *Alternative Therapies in Health and Medicine* 9, no. 2 (March/April 2003): 20–21.

traindications, respected hospitals—among them the NIH's Warren Grant Magnuson Clinical Center, New York–Presbyterian Hospital/Columbia University Medical Center, Yale–New Haven Hospital, Memorial Sloan-Kettering Cancer Center, Dana-Farber/Harvard Cancer Center, George Washington University Hospital, and the University of Texas M. D. Anderson Cancer Center—have gone ahead. As researcher Gala True, Ph.D., says, "Science needs to catch up to the demands of patients."

Fourteen

REIKI AND INTEGRATIVE MEDICINE

Wherever the art of medicine is loved, there is also a love of humanity.

HIPPOCRATES

Health care is in an unprecendented period of change, and policy can vary widely not only from locale to locale but also, in large hospitals, from department to department. Let's step back and take a look at what is happening in health care and how Reiki might fit.

Conventional medicine, complementary and alternative medicine, integrative medicine, and *traditional medicine*. These are terms that are bandied about by health-care professionals and consumers—and are often used in conflicting and misleading ways. Understanding these terms will help make sense of current, evolving shifts in health care in the United States and how these changes will affect the ways you can access Reiki.

CONVENTIONAL MEDICINE

Conventional, or mainstream, medicine is currently the dominant medical system in the United States. Also referred to as biomedicine, it is based on biomedical research science and largely consists of "medical" diagnostic techniques and interventions such as blood tests, scans, surgery, and medication. Because research is continually shedding light on the efficacy of newly studied approaches, medical science is constantly evolving, and approaches once thought to be unscientific—including lifestyle changes involving exercise, stress management, and nutrition—are increasingly incorporated into mainstream treatment.

COMPLEMENTARY AND ALTERNATIVE MEDICINE (CAM)

Those approaches, techniques, or medical systems not considered to be sufficiently validated by scientific research are relegated to the status of "unproven" and are termed "alternative" (if used instead of standard medical practices) or "complementary" (if used in addition to them). They are largely derived from indigenous medical traditions.

For quite some time, these approaches were referred to as "fringe" by conventional physicians, medical schools, and research institutions, with the inherent assumption that they were useless at best and possibly dangerous. That perception began to change in 1993 when a Harvard research team led by David Eisenberg, M.D., published a phone survey of health-care practices in the prestigious medical journal the *New England Journal of Medicine*.[1] Thirty-four percent of those responding to the survey had used at least one of the sixteen listed CAM therapies in the past year. Seven years later, in his follow-up study, that percentage had increased significantly to 42 percent.[2] CAM therapies were commonly used by people with chronic conditions, including back problems, anxiety, depression, and headaches. What was particularly shocking to the conventional health-care industry was that Americans paid more out of pocket for this care ($21.2 billion in 1997, with at least $12.2 billion paid out of pocket) than they did for out-of-pocket hospital expenses; that they usually didn't tell their physicians; and that most patients used conventional, scientific medicine and traditional remedies such as herbs, acupuncture, and Reiki *at the same time.*

Eisenberg was the first to publish these findings but not the only academic looking at the situation. Researchers want to know who, how many, and why? Science had drawn a line between health care and lifestyle (a distinction that research is blurring). But such a division never even existed in the paradigm of holistic healing, with its focus on healthful living and prevention, making it impossible to precisely separate out who is using complementary therapies. For example, adding prayer specifically for health to the list of therapies utilized greatly increases the percentage of users.[3] The common use of prayer for health is interesting in view of studies that show that patients use complementary therapies because these approaches fit their values[4] and that people choosing unconventional health-care practitioners score higher on psychospiritual measures than those who choose conventional doctors.[5] Other studies have shown that even seniors seek care from complementary practitioners, usually when conventional medicine does not bring relief from chronic problems.[6]

Patients are disgruntled with the dehumanization of medicine, skyrocketing costs, and loss of control through managed care, matters that also trouble many medical professionals. Physicians have become concerned with such things as the overuse of antibiotics, unnecessary diagnostic testing, and the increasing threat of litigation. Looking to get out of the war zone that biomedicine too often becomes, many physicians seek gentler, more satisfying ways to practice medicine and interact with patients. With increasing pressure both from within the profession and from patients, conventional medicine has begun to recognize that CAM therapies have a place in health care, offering patients something not available through standardized medical care alone.

There are some nonemergency ailments for which patients seek relief using therapies as alternatives to more invasive medical procedures—a course of acupuncture treatments rather than back surgery, for example. More and more often, patients use therapies like these simultaneously with medical care to support well-being and to mitigate the side effects of pharmaceuticals and medical procedures. This supportive role is of particular value to conventional medicine if it means patients can more easily sustain arduous conventional medical and surgical therapies and recover faster from illness and surgery.

Leading professionals in both conventional medicine and CAM recognize that the patient who is receiving care from both perspectives is probably receiving better care. The hope is that collaboration between practitioners of conventional medicine and traditional healing therapies will create a broader, more humanistic approach to health care.

INTEGRATIVE MEDICINE

A holistic approach to health care that incorporates traditional healing approaches with conventional medicine has been dubbed "integrative medicine." This relationship-centered approach often involves a health-care team that not only addresses illness, but also gives patients tools and motivation to strengthen their well-being. Integrative medicine engages patients in decision making and collaborative self-care both preventively and when treatment is needed. Integrative medicine honors the dictum *First do no harm* that is valued by conventional and traditional practitioners alike by championing the use of less invasive, low-cost interventions before resorting to the heroic measures so readily used in hospitals today. An integrative approach honors the patient's needs, means, and preferences.

As Andrew Weil, M.D., author of *Healthy Aging* and popular and sage champion of health-care reform, points out, we'll know how successfully integrative medicine has taken hold when we no longer see qualifiers like "conventional," "traditional," or even "integrative" used. When integrative medicine has become standard practice, we'll have good medicine for everyone.

Conventional medicine often cites the paucity of research as an obstacle to integrating traditional therapies into standard care. Given the relative safety of most CAM therapies and science's dismal track record in protecting the public from real dangers, this perspective just doesn't make sense. I remember the thalidomide scandal when I was a kid—babies born with birth defects because their mothers had been prescribed the drug during pregnancy. And what about DES? That both these drugs were given to pregnant women is unconscionable. More recently, we have seen such widespread tragedies as the cover-up of data linking the pain medication Vioxx to heart attack and stroke, and the discovery that antidepressants effective in adults can agitate teens to the point of suicide (the drugs were never tested on teens).

Meanwhile, how many double-blind studies were run on quadruple-bypass surgery before it was used? None. In fact, bypass surgery was practiced for thirteen years before being studied. Although everyone would like to see more research, the clinical practice of medicine is not as tightly linked to research as some scientists pretend.[7] The problem is not so much an underwhelming body of research to support CAM as it is a lack of education.* Physicians feel more comfortable innovating when using familiar tools in a paradigm they understand and trust. Until doctors are taught the paradigm of natural, holistic medicine from which traditional healing therapies are derived, how can they be comfortable using these therapies? Once physicians understand the logic behind traditional, nonscientific therapies, they will be able to guide patients more skillfully and realistically in integrating these therapies into health care.

TRADITIONAL MEDICINE

Traditional medical systems such as Ayurveda from India, Chinese medicine, and Tibetan medicine, while not based on modern science, are nonetheless based on

---

*CAM survey courses are increasingly available in medical schools, but a more comprehensive education is needed for physicians to be more than pidgin conversant in this area. The Program in Integrative Medicine (PIM) at the University of Arizona encourages doctors to actually experience various CAMs, learn some basic skills, and create working relationships with credible practitioners. Two medical texts that specifically address Reiki are *Kaplan and Sadock's Synopsis of Psychiatry: Behavioral Sciences, Clinical Psychiatry,* by Benjamin James Sadock, M.D., and Virginia Alcott Sadock, M.D., (p. 865) and *Complementary Therapies in Rehabilitation: Evidence for Efficacy in Therapy, Prevention, and Wellness,* by Carol Davis, Ph.D. (chapter 14).

observation and logic. There is nothing magical about these medical systems, although the results may appear magical to someone who doesn't understand the mechanism of action. For example, despite having been used for thousands of years, acupuncture seemed implausible to conventional doctors who lacked an understanding of Chinese medicine. While medical science might remain unconvinced of Chinese medical theory, there is increasing evidence of acupuncture's efficacy. Not yet able to document how acupuncture works, researchers are testing it in a variety of applications. There is good evidence that acupuncture works for nausea and vomiting, facial pain, dental pain, and knee pain from osteoarthritis, and some evidence that it works for back pain, neck pain, and headache, but science is unable to say simply that acupuncture works.

This brings us to an important difference between traditional medical systems and biomedicine. Because traditional medical systems do not rely exclusively on outer verification but also employ finely tuned intuitive skills, they anticipate breakthroughs in understanding and knowledge. Advances in traditional therapeutics build upon existing knowledge rather than reversing it. This is in sharp contrast to scientific medicine, where the latest advance often undermines or contradicts the last thing learned.

From an indigenous medical perspective, strengthening existing well-being is primary; the best way to treat disease is to prevent it. An early Chinese medical text, *The Yellow Emperor's Classic of Medicine,* expresses it thus: "Treating illness after it has begun is like suppressing revolt after it has broken out. If someone digs a well when thirsty, or forges weapons after becoming engaged in battle, one cannot help but ask: Are these actions not too late?"[8]

The knowledge available in other indigenous systems that have not become as systematized, such as African and Native American medicine, is still surprisingly sophisticated. When used by a knowledgeable practitioner, traditional therapies can be as valuable with contemporary scourges as they are with more common diseases. For example, Michael Smith, M.D., an acupuncturist at Lincoln Recovery Center in the Bronx, New York, was able to support people with AIDS before the disease was even identified by the Centers for Disease Control. Asian medicine identifies dysfunction in the system and seeks to restore balance, so Smith was able to address areas of weakened functioning without knowing the invading pathogens. Traditional Chinese medicine's treatment goals are always multidimensional, seeking to effect symptom relief, immune enhancement, and in this application, a reduction of side effects from medication.

Conventional medicine, on the other hand, is reductionist and focused on disease. It looks at illness in ever-increasing degrees of specificity and targets cures that can be applied across a widely varying population of patients. Although the World Health Organization (WHO) has recognized good health as more than the absence of disease, conventional medicine's focus on disease has kept it from developing a model for health. And because no one experiences himself as a collection of discrete body parts Velcroed together that can be disassembled, replaced, and reassembled until the warranty runs out, this poses a problem.

Traditional medical approaches are holistic, addressing every aspect of the patient's being—body, mind, and spirit—functioning as a complex system. Traditional approaches care for the patient first, recognizing the uniqueness of the individual, and addressing disease within the context of the particular individual experiencing it. Understanding that healing comes from within, traditional medicine seeks to enhance overall well-being, thereby enabling the patient to address illness more effectively. Rather than reducing the patient to organs—or even cells—in isolation, holistic approaches consider not only the entire person but also how she functions as part of a greater whole, socially, culturally, and spiritually. Where holistic medicine seeks to engage and strengthen the body's ability to heal, conventional medicine often replaces or overrides the malfunction without addressing the underlying issue.

From a traditional perspective—for example, the perspective of those Americans, especially but not exclusively recent immigrants, who have never fully adopted conventional medicine, preferring to rely on traditional ways to avoid or cope with illness—conventional Western medicine can look clumsy and shortsighted, like patching the crack on the third-floor ceiling without taking into account that the foundation is sinking. These people may or may not eventually go to a physician, but they don't run to the doctor for every sore throat or ache and pain. A lot of their health care comes as part of what physicians call lifestyle choices—everyday interventions as mundane as adapting diet to the changing seasons, for example, or reaching for ginger or garlic or even schnapps to warm the body after getting chilled.

These traditionalists weren't impressed when science decided that getting chilled doesn't make you sick. Their experience and common sense told them getting chilled is unbalancing, and when one's system is off balance, it doesn't function optimally and it's easier to get sick. This population would often seek health care from a trusted member of the community, sometimes called a barefoot doctor.

On the other hand, it would be naive—if not foolhardy—to ignore the technological advances of modern medicine in favor of a natural, less effective approach, once a disease process has progressed. Such an either/or perspective is potentially dangerous and completely unnecessary since these approaches can be skillfully combined.

THE PROMISE OF
COLLABORATIVE MEDICINE

Although it may not be apparent how such divergent perspectives could be anything but oppositional, when used skillfully in conjunction, these approaches can not only support one another but also deliver the best possible care to the patient. For example, conventional medicine offers insulin injections to replace the insulin that the pancreas is not secreting in diabetics. No one would argue that this is anything less than a great achievement of modern science. But what if we combined insulin treatment with therapies such as Reiki, which appears to balance the endocrine system and might lessen the need for insulin or slow the progression of the disease and its complications? Such an innovative approach becomes more desirable as diseases, such as adult-onset diabetes, that were once seen only in adults begin showing up in childhood. A medical repair or stopgap measure that could keep an adult functioning for years longer may not work so well when started in childhood (of course, the ultimate holistic medicine would seek to understand why the *overall* health of our nation is declining).

The irony is that these traditional medical systems, which often have many centuries of use and experience behind them, become confused by the public with less sound New Age practices. Not only do traditional medical approaches adhere to the Hippocratic admonition *First, do no harm,* but traditional approaches are by definition *more conservative* than conventional medicine, using the least invasive methods possible while building the patient's overall strength and well-being. As Lao Tzu expounded over 2,500 years ago, *Better a foot behind than an inch ahead,* meaning the skilled practitioner does as little as possible to enable the person to improve. Traditional medical systems appreciate that the most direct way is not necessarily the best way for the patient's overall, long-term well-being.

HEALING, WITH OR WITHOUT CURE

Conventional health care tends to focus on disease management and cure. Healing and the maintenance of general well-being are not usually emphasized, especially in managed-care plans. But anyone with a health challenge knows that both cure and healing are valuable. Since they do not automatically occur together, and we may have to find them in different places, it is useful to understand the distinction between the two.

Cure is objective and disease-specific. We are dependent on specialists and technology to confirm if and when we can be cured of anything more complex than a cold or flu. But we can be certified "cured" and still be far from healthy. Patients often feel left out of the process of cure, passive and distressed, and this does not bode well for medical outcomes. In the worst-case scenario, people actually die of aggressive attempts to cure. Clearly cure is not desirable in and of itself, but only in the context of overall health and well-being. This is where healing comes in.

Healing involves the alignment of our body, mind, and spirit. It addresses the places where our lives are in our own hands. There is no affidavit that guarantees healing. Healing is subjective and requires our active participation.

HEALING ON HER OWN TERMS

Helen told me right away that she'd come for Reiki only to please her employer, an accountant who had long been a client of mine. He hated watching a valued employee struggle and offered to finance her Reiki sessions. Free treatment or not, Helen wasn't much interested in what I had to offer. She sat erect and proud on my treatment table that warm September afternoon, a slender, comely sixty-five-year-old wincing slightly from the pain of her third recurrence of cancer, which had metastasized from her lungs to her liver and now to her spine. Locking eyes with me, she said in her raspy, defiant voice, "I'm not a good candidate for this kind of thing. I don't want to quit smoking, and I'm not going to change my diet."

I loved her feistiness and decided to match it in kind. "That's good," I said, "because I'm not going to ask you to quit smoking or to change your diet." I paused strategically before adding, "I'm not even going to ask you to live."

The spark in her eyes told me I had her. Even at her age, no one had yet supported her right to choose. I continued, "Maybe there's something else I can do for you. Maybe you're afraid of pain, or maybe you'll just want to come back because you like me so much. Why don't we do a treatment and then you can tell me what, if anything, I can do for you."

Her dry lips cracked a smile as she carefully lay down. An hour later, she was surprised by how peaceful and refreshed she felt.

"What do you want?" I asked her once she had sat upright.

Helen took a deep breath. "I *am* afraid of the pain," she admitted, "but mostly I want to be with my daughter when she gives birth to our first grandchild at the holidays. They live in Oregon. And"—she looked at me hard—"I have to keep working till then to keep my medical benefits, which I need." I told her I thought we could achieve those goals—if we worked together regularly. She came every week for treatment, spent a month on the West Coast at the holidays and met her grandchild—and died peacefully at home in her sleep the following May.

Cure was never Helen's goal. Although it looked to me as if she still had a lot to live for, she showed no interest in cure, or even long-term management of the cancer that was taking over her body. But she expressed clearly that she wanted healing.

Helen had to reach outside the health-care system for Reiki healing, and she was fortunate to be able to do so. However, it is sometimes possible to find Reiki within the system.

TEACHING REIKI IN A HOSPITAL SETTING

In 1995, Robert Schmehr, CSW, learned of the Reiki classes I was offering at Gay Men's Health Crisis (GMHC). Schmehr was then a psychotherapist at the HIV clinic at New York City's Beth Israel Medical Center. The administration had just green-lighted his vision to support conventional HIV care with complementary therapies such as Reiki. By this time, patients were beginning highly active antiretroviral therapy (HAART) and struggling with side effects. It was hoped that teaching outpatients to practice Reiki self-treatment would give them a tool to improve their quality of life. Classes began in January 1997 after an initial presentation to staff.

Inner-city HIV clinics such as this one provide care primarily for a disenfranchised segment of our society, people who have weak family ties and social support and who are ill equipped to navigate the bureaucracy of government support programs. Many patients come with multiple diagnoses, including psychiatric ones. Histories of substance abuse, homelessness, and incarceration are common. Injection drug use is the primary risk factor for HIV infection for about three-quarters of the clinic's patients. Some of my Reiki students at Beth Israel were diagnosed with mental illnesses ranging from anxiety and depression to psychotic conditions that were managed well enough to enable them to be in a group program.

The classes were held on four successive days, and patients began practicing Reiki immediately. Interest in the program spread as the Beth Israel staff witnessed the benefits

Reiki brought their patients. As in the classes at GMHC, the physical changes reported by the students included relief from chronic pain, headaches, and body aches, and improved sleep and digestion. Physicians and psychiatrists at Beth Israel saw another dimension of benefit in their patients who practiced Reiki: Patients' moods, coping skills, and overall functioning improved, and their relationship with their health-care providers became stronger as the patients became better partners in their health care. Schmehr noted this as a valued gain in a clinic that specialized in making its program user-friendly for people who traditionally had difficulty obtaining high-quality health-care services.

"Reiki is an important tool to help patients create safety," said Schmehr. He and other mental health professionals at the clinic noted growth in the self-awareness of patients who practiced Reiki. "As patients become more self-aware," he observed, "they have healthier options for managing stress and pain." Many patients specifically reported using Reiki self-treatment to help them stay sober and off drugs. Some patients who were self-motivated to reduce their psychiatric medications used Reiki to lower the dosage or wean themselves completely, supervised by their psychiatrist. Other patients, who had been irregular in taking needed medications, gained a new self-awareness, which helped them recognize their need for psychiatric medications, and they became more motivated to take their meds regularly.[9]

According to Schmehr, "The Reiki class moved the health-care dialogue to a new level." And, for those patients who were distrustful of conventional medicine, Reiki was "like an olive branch." He felt that the practice let the patients know the staff cared for them—and the patients began trusting the staff. It was a powerful statement to the patients to be offered a nonauthoritarin educational opportunity in the context of a medical setting.

I learned so much teaching these classes. One thing I came to understand was that even at that time, there were already many physicians who were sincerely interested in complementary therapies but who couldn't see their way past the huge cultural divide. Once I began teaching in the hospital, I was seen as "legitimate," and physicians approached me with questions and often a desire to learn Reiki. I appreciated their frustration. They wanted to offer their patients more support, but didn't know how to obtain the help that might be available outside the system. These physicians didn't know how to identify a good holistic practitioner, and they didn't know how to speak to one if they found one. They recognized the language and cultural differences, and they were stumped how to bridge the gap. But the doctors had observed positive changes in their patients who used Reiki, and they wanted to know more.

The classes in the HIV clinics (Schmehr later made them available also in the HIV clinics at St. Luke's and Roosevelt hospitals) were for patients only, so physicians began coming to my Reiki classes outside the hospital. They practiced on themselves, and many brought moments of Reiki into their routine medical care. Because Reiki can make an immediate and palpable difference, it can help patients and physicians alike find a way to healing, to reach for wholeness, even in the strict confines of biomedicine.

A patient at the Morningside Clinic at St. Luke's, Michel arrived from the Gold Coast just in time to be diagnosed with AIDS. He spoke French and understood some English. I did my best to underline the important points in French, we had an occasional translator, and we connected through Reiki. At the end of the class, Michel said, "Now when I look in the mirror, I see that I am not alone."

REIKI CAN BENEFIT
ANY TREATMENT PLAN

Is Reiki all one ever needs? Common sense tells us no. There is nothing that fills all needs all the time. Even when in vibrant health, a good night's sleep doesn't save us from the need for good food and company and mental stimulation. The more unhealthy the person, the more likely other treatment will be needed.

Although Reiki is rarely all a patient needs, this gentle healing practice can fill an important need in health care, facilitating the diagnostic phase and the delivery of conventional care. Reiki's harmonizing, relaxing influence seems to set the stage for more effective care and higher satisfaction on the part of patient and caregiver. Reiki provides near-immediate stress reduction. A calmer, more centered patient is not only easier to care for—and safer to study with invasive tests such as IVP (intravenous pyelogram), MRI, and bone-marrow biopsy—but also more likely to become engaged in the process of care. Recipients of Reiki report a sense of bonding with the practitioner, and third-party, non-Reiki care providers have observed that Reiki seems to enhance rapport between patient and medical caregivers.

Reiki seems to prime the patient for healing, no matter what biomedical intervention is needed. And Reiki sends up no red flags to medical caregivers; there are no known contraindications, no time when Reiki is dangerous. Indeed, Reiki adds a healing dimension to even the most invasive tests or treatments such as bone-marrow biopsy or surgery.

People typically report feeling comforted by even brief Reiki treatment, and many patients attribute accelerated recovery times to Reiki. It has been shown effective in the management of anxiety and pain, and may make it possible to reduce medications. Lewis Mehl-Madrona, M.D., Ph.D., and Native American healing elder, has been integrating complementary therapies and native practices with conventional medicine for twenty-five years. Even before I trained him to practice Reiki, this accomplished physician/healer observed, "Once Reiki is added to the treatment plan, all the other interventions being used seem to work better." Reiki can gently change the patient's consciousness, redirecting his attention toward wellness. Traditional medicine considers this shift in consciousness necessary if there is to be any lasting improvement.

I've often wondered what difference it might make if moments of Reiki were available to patients waiting in doctors' offices and emergency rooms. Even those unfamiliar with Reiki's particular benefits can appreciate that having someone who is focused on the patient's well-being offer him noninvasive, gentle attention is probably a plus. The patient getting more attention generally does better than the patient getting less.

WHAT ARE THE OPTIONS FOR INTEGRATIVE CARE?

Integrative medical care is available from a wide spectrum of venues ranging from very-scientific-with-some-comfort care to a lifestyle-centered, only-call-the-doctor-when-needed approach. Each patient has to choose which of the options available in his area best meets his needs and preferences. The time spent researching the possibilities and interviewing caregivers is time well spent. Best to do it now, to strengthen your well-being so that when a health concern arises, you already have a team in place.

A growing number of hospitals are responding to consumer demand by including complementary therapies in the menu of services available to patients. If you receive your health care at a clinic, find out what is available and let the staff know what you are looking for. Medicine is a business, and many clinics have added Reiki and other therapies in response to patient demand.

Patients can also receive care from medical and complementary-care providers at private outpatient integrative medical centers. Often, care is supervised by a physician who refers to other practitioners on staff as needed; but sometimes care is provided by primarily conventional doctors who have learned a few CAM "tricks," so be sure to ask exactly how each center you investigate is organized. The staff may or may not have patient conferences during which they collaborate on cases.

There are also primary-care physicians whose skills and training are primarily conventional but who practice integrative medicine by referring patients to local complementary practitioners. These physicians may be more or less knowledgeable about nonmedical care options, but they understand the role these therapies play in health care and they have a network of trusted local practitioners. Having the combined care of an open-minded conventional physician and seasoned traditional healers in whatever arrangement is available provides health care from a broad perspective and depth of experience.

There are also patients who prefer to manage their health care themselves. They often receive the bulk of their care from nonmedical practitioners and consult their physician on an as-needed basis.

Take time not only to investigate your local options but also to learn about yourself as a patient so that you know which situation will best support you. Do you call your doctor at the first sneeze, or do you visit your acupuncturist like clockwork at the turn of the seasons? Are you passive or interactive with your primary-care provider? Do you think of your doctor as an authority or an expert collaborator?

It is not reasonable to assume that you will get the best complementary care at a conventional medical center, where the appreciation of complementary therapies may be filtered through a decidedly medical value system or where they may be added only for the cachet. You have to read between the lines. For example, a hospital website that states that all practitioners should be licensed obviously subscribes to the conventional medical hierarchy (most complementary therapies do not have licensing). Another hospital website advises patients to check that the practitioner is willing to communicate with the oncologist, but it is more likely the oncologist who is unavailable or uninterested in this conversation. That said, if you feel safe receiving care only in a medical environment, honor that preference.

REIKI AND MEDICAL INSURANCE

As of this writing, the only way Reiki is covered by insurance is when it is included as part of a reimbursable treatment such as physical therapy, massage, or palliative care or delivered by a nurse or licensed health-care professional as part of routine care. According to James Dillard, M.D., medical director for Complementary and Alternative Medicine at Oxford Health Plans of United Health Group, it is unlikely that insurance will ever cover Reiki. Rather, Dillard advises consumers to look into the availability of medical savings accounts (MSAs) at their workplaces. There are several types of MSAs: health savings accounts (HSAs), flexible spending accounts (FSAs), and health reimbursement accounts (HRAs). Each is a specific variation of a new strategy to help relieve the burden of health-care costs by setting aside pretax dollars for health-care-related expenditures. The definition of acceptable expenses varies, so be sure to research which is the best choice for your needs and verify that Reiki is an allowable expense. Dillard sees this as the most likely scenario in which Reiki would be covered.

REIKI AND LAW

Each state creates its own laws governing health-care practice. Additionally, there may be local laws that impact on health-care delivery, such as laws restricting the practice of Reiki or even massage. Many state legislatures have not caught up with the current trend toward including complementary and alternative therapies in health care. The good news is that generally the letter of outdated law is not being followed.

Although Reiki is widely deemed to be noninvasive, there are still areas where professional Reiki practice might run into legal snafus (I have not heard of any concerns about students practicing at home). Consumers and professionals who are concerned about the legalities of practice in their area need to inform themselves of local ordinances and state laws. Legal advice, like medical advice, is beyond the scope of this book and is not its intention. Rather, I'd like to broadly frame the situation so that readers who wish to research these matters have a foundation from which to do so. As you read, please keep in mind that health-care choices are also spiritual choices. When it comes to entrusting our lives and the lives of those we love to the care of another, we choose what we believe in, what is real to us, within our financial means. Laws that limit our ability to choose according to our beliefs and our values when it matters most need to be looked at very carefully.

State laws define and license the practice of medicine. The definition of the medical practice is broad enough in most states to include all the healing arts. Some health-care services are specifically exempt. For example, as long as nurses practice within the scope of the nursing statute, they are not vulnerable to charges of practicing medicine without a license. However, the practice of a therapy such as Reiki for which no state licensing exists could be interpreted to fall under the jurisdiction of the broadly defined legal practice of medicine. Unlicensed health-care practitioners could thus technically be vulnerable to being charged with practicing medicine without a license. So why not license Reiki the way acupuncture is licensed?

Licensing law is meant to protect the public from unskilled practitioners of modalities that are understood to carry risk. Because Reiki is largely practiced as home self-care and is universally deemed to be noninvasive and to carry no risk, it is unlikely that any state legislature would spend the time and money required to create licensing for Reiki practice. But without a specific legal exemption, Reiki practice could fall under the legal definition of medical practice.

Additionally, Reiki may be included under massage licensing law in state or local ordinances. As of this writing, these states which regulate massage do not include Reiki under massage regulations as long as Reiki only is being practiced: Alabama, Delaware, Hawaii, Louisiana, Maine, Maryland, Missouri, New York, New Hampshire, New Mexico, North Carolina, Texas, Utah, and West Virginia. These states do not regulate massage or Reiki: Arkansas, California, Colorado, Kansas, Michigan, Minnesota, Montana, Oklahoma, Pennsylvania, Vermont, and Wyoming. The Florida Board of Massage Therapy has issued an interpretation specifically requiring Reiki practitioners to have massage licenses. Massachusetts and Indiana are states in transition. Because the legal situation is evolving, it's vital that professionals stay current.

In 2000, Minnesota responded to a grassroots movement by passing a landmark health-care freedom bill that decriminalized the practice of low-risk unlicensed health-care practices. The new Minnesota law exempts practitioners from criminal charges of practicing medicine without a license as long as they do not participate in a detailed list of prohibited behaviors such as: puncturing the skin, administering prescription drugs or controlled substances, providing a medical diagnosis, and more. Practitioners are also mandated to provide clients with a customized notice form called the Client Bill of Rights, letting clients know they are not licensed by the state as health-care practitioners, what their education and training is, and what the nature or basic theory of their practice is. Although practitioners are not required to sign up with the government before they practice, the state has set up an office to handle complaints about such practitioners.

Minnesota attorney Diane Miller worked with the Minnesota Natural Health–Legal Reform Project, a group of determined health-freedom advocates, to draft the original bill and work as one of its chief advocates. Since then, Rhode Island, California and Louisiana have created their own version of health-care freedom, and nine states introduced similar legislation. Twenty-five more states are now moving in that direction. All this is a response to grassroots activism. Since medical law varies so much from state to state, state law must be researched in each state, and the particular points negotiated according to the popular issues being championed and the political climate in the state's capitol. Oklahoma and Idaho have historically been free states for unlicensed practitioners.

Diane Miller founded National Health Freedom Action (NHFA), www .national healthfreedom.org, to support grassroots organizers in other states. NHFA is a strong advocate for state jurisdiction over health-care-practice issues and works to protect the rights of the state to protect its citizens. They support broad-based consumer access to all health-care options and work to protect the diversity within and among state health-care cultures. NHFA sees the state practice laws as an avenue to encourage innovation in health care.

Physicians may be understandably concerned about liability when integrating complementary or alternative-healing approaches such as Reiki into their medical practice, or even when asked by patients to comment on such therapies. Michael H. Cohen, Esq., is at the forefront of this new field of CAM law. In a paper published in the peer-reviewed medical journal *Annals of Internal Medicine,* Cohen and his coauthor, David Eisenberg M.D., both of Harvard Medical School, offered a commonsense guide for physicians to consider when recommending a therapy that lies outside conventional practice. They suggest getting the answers to two questions:

Is the therapy safe?

Is the therapy effective?

If the therapy is safe and effective, there is no reason not to recommend it, according to Cohen and Eisenberg. Reiki is widely considered safe, but researchers are just beginning to investigate its effectiveness. Physicians who have firsthand experience of Reiki may feel confident in recommending Reiki, and the growing number of hospitals where Reiki is offered indicates that this is a common assessment. However, for physicians who agree that Reiki (or any other CAM therapy) is safe but remain unconvinced of its effectiveness, Cohen and Eisenberg suggest tolerance of their patients' use of that therapy.[10] Cohen's website, www.camlawblog.com, is an invaluable resource.

REIKI AND PUBLIC HEALTH

Reiki is deeply healing to those who have been traumatized in any way—rape, crime, war, terror, or torture. Reiki treatment quickly reconnects people with their sense of wholeness, without any talking, without disrobing, and with either the lightest touch or off the body, as needed. As demonstrated in the HIV classes discussed earlier, Reiki can also address the special needs of the underserved, helping to empower disenfranchised populations such as the urban poor and the homeless, giving them not only a tool with which to help themselves, but a practice to transform their sense of self.

Lincoln Recovery Center is an intensive outpatient chemical dependency program in the Bronx where Michael Smith, M.D., has been the medical and administrative director for thirty years. Successful addiction treatment involves clients in taking responsibility for their own lives. Reiki has been available there since 2001, when an addictions counselor began incorporating Reiki into services. Reiki treatment was particularly welcome in the battered-women's program. Eventually some of the clients asked to be trained as practitioners. Once trained in First Degree Reiki, the women began volunteering in the domestic violence shelters where they had once stayed.

The Center offers separate support groups for men and women, so that battered women will not feel intimidated to express themselves. When a women's Reiki group had to be moved to the men's floor, however, the men's group, including the very tough-minded counselor, became intrigued by what the women were doing. The men wanted treatment, but the request brought many questions. Would the women be able to reach out to these men who might have attitudes toward them? Would they have to explain what they were doing? Most important, was it possible for this to be a transforming experience? The women practitioners agreed to offer chair Reiki, and it was readily apparent that this was a transforming experience for all. It was not necessary to speak about Reiki at all, just to do it.

Bringing Reiki into Conventional Medical Settings

The Reiki program at Portsmouth Regional Hospital in New Hampshire is thriving with a full-time lay Reiki master and has spurred the creation of Reiki programs in other hospitals in the area. Nonetheless, it is a rare hospital administrator who has the vision to create such a program or to hire a lay Reiki master to give treatment and train staff.

I have created various kinds of Reiki programs in a number of New York City hospitals and have interviewed or consulted with others around the country. The vision and standards for integration vary enormously from setting to setting, and in large city hospitals, they can vary even from department to department. Plans to create Reiki programs can get bogged down in bureaucratic complexity that's impossible to untangle.

In view of this, the most promising way at this time to integrate Reiki into most conventional settings is to train existing staff. Targeting personnel in emergency rooms, surgery, pain and palliative care services, and hospice settings would deliver Reiki to the places where its benefits are most obvious. This is, in fact, what happened at the NIH's Clinical Center in Bethesda, Maryland. Two staff members, a massage therapist and a chaplain, were already Reiki practitioners. As they integrated Reiki into their care with good results, other staff became interested. Trainings for staff were organized, and Reiki was soon added to the services menu.

Because medical centers are entrenched in the conventional approach rather than using more holistic practices, John Graham-Pole, M.D., says that often the best way to introduce Reiki is for physicians and other health caregivers simply "to use it ourselves and encourage others to do so" by introducing it in presentations and when training medical students.

Many physicians I've trained comment on how easily Reiki bridges the gap that can exist between touch that is investigative and touch that is therapeutic. Sezelle Gereau Haddon, M.D., is a pediatric ear, nose, and throat surgeon at Children's Hospital and at the Continuum Center for Health and Healing in New York City. She finds that Reiki seamlessly turns the moments of touch that initiate a physical exam into moments of healing. Touch can carry many implications and has to be appropriate to be beneficial.[11] Because Reiki touch is generally offered through clothing, and because patients typically experience it as comforting, physicians find moments to access Reiki that fall well within the parameters of appropriate touch.

A licensed acupuncturist and chiropractor before training as a physician, James Dillard, M.D., uses a plethora of conventional and CAM techniques. He strongly advocates health-care professionals having broad skills. Since most hospitals are not yet hiring Reiki practitioners to offer treatment to patients, Dillard sees "the seamless integration from dually and triply trained practitioners as a good way to bring Reiki to patients for whom it might not otherwise be available."

If you want to bring Reiki into a conventional care setting, look at the individual situation to identify those caregivers who are interested and whose duties allow for such integration. Dillard says, "When you have ministers working in palliative care settings for years and you train them as Reiki practitioners, they can easily add that to what they are doing at the bedside. What a fabulous combination—they have the access and the time." Patients who respond with interest to their Reiki experience can be referred to local Reiki practitioners for treatment or training.

REIKI IN MEDICAL EDUCATION

A powerful way to bring Reiki into hospitals and other conventional medical settings is to educate medical students. I have presented Reiki at many medical schools and trained medical students, residents and fellows at the Program in Integrative Medicine at the University of Arizona.[12] The students always show avid interest. Often it is they who create the opportunity. Even more effective than teaching them about Reiki is to train medical students to actually practice. The experience of supporting themselves with Reiki through their years of rigorous training gives them profound insight into the process of healing as well as a valuable clinical tool. And as we empower the doctors of tomorrow with this spiritual healing practice, we increase the likelihood that they will wield the power of medical technology within a context of humanistic medicine.

Many medical schools have recently established wellness programs that give their students an opportunity to learn traditional healing practices such as meditation, yoga, qigong, and Reiki. I teach First Degree Reiki as part of the wellness program at the Albert Einstein College of Medicine, under the leadership of the associate dean for Educational Affairs, Albert S. Kuperman, Ph.D. He says, "Our expectation is that by experiencing the beneficial effects of these methods on their own health and well-being, medical students will come to appreciate their value as adjuncts to conventional medicine in prevention and healing in their future patients."

PREPARING REIKI PROFESSIONALS FOR MEDICAL COLLABORATION

It's truly wonderful that physicians, nurses, and allied health-care professionals are practicing Reiki on themselves and integrating moments of Reiki into routine health care. Many times, these Reiki-trained medical professionals are the catalysts for bringing Reiki into a health-care setting in a more formal way. Their contribution is vital, yet there is only so much they can do—unless they want to give up their day jobs. Offering full Reiki treatments to patient after patient, day after day, including staff as is possible, requires a level of expertise different from that required for integrating moments of Reiki into medical care. And staff and patient Reiki training can be done only by a Reiki master. Be cautious about taking on the role of Reiki expert at your workplace. You may find yourself quickly overwhelmed. Especially if you want to create a Reiki program where you work, be it hospital, hospice, nursing home, or outpatient care center, I suggest finding a Reiki professional appropriate for medical collaboration and bringing that practitioner aboard as early as possible.

If you are thinking of becoming a Reiki professional, remember that the three levels of Reiki training, even when given the traditional way, with substantial class time and breaks between levels to practice, prepares the student to practice Reiki, but not professionally. If you want to be a Reiki professional, find a way to log in hours and hours of treatment, preferably supervised, or at least find mentoring. In every field, professionals are trained by other professionals. Why would Reiki be different?

Reiki practitioners who wish to collaborate in medical environments would do well with even more training. First of all, learn medical boundaries—how to speak to a patient in a health-care setting without violating laws of confidentiality or breaching medical practice. Educate yourself on the fundamentals of the biomedical health-care environment, how it functions, how medical professionals communicate with one another. Learn what concerns physicians so that you can intelligently address those concerns. Learn how to document treatments. And if you want to collaborate on research, learn the scientific method and study some of the many papers written about the challenges of creating viable research on CAM modalities. You don't have to be a researcher, but you want to be able to enter the conversation. Medical Reiki practitioners really don't need to learn anatomy and physiology. It's not relevant to Reiki practice.

Most important, medical Reiki practitioners need to develop their own ways of expressing Reiki practice that are clear, concise, logical, and at the same time reflective of their individual experience and understanding—all that without making any claims. Although it's helpful to know a little medical language, even if it's just in order not to feel intimidated, remember that health-care staff don't want you to be a medical professional—they are interested in your experience; they simply need to be able to understand what you're saying as you share it. Develop opportunities to speak about Reiki to people you don't expect to be particularly interested. Always include moments of hands-on Reiki, and then learn from their questions and feedback.

I offer classes in a variety of formats, including teleclasses, to help interested Reiki practitioners prepare themselves for professional practice and for medical collaboration, whether they want to work in hospitals, hospice, nursing homes, adult day care or other care facilities, or with private practice physicians. These classes are open to Reiki practitioners at any level and from any practice style who want to develop their ability to communicate Reiki credibly. We discuss how and why Reiki is already being used in conventional medicine and how to interact effectively with physicians through understanding medical culture, professional standards, and clinical skills. Depending on the needs of the particular class, there is an introduction to medical research: an overview of the scientific method, the specific challenges of Reiki research, and an update on published Reiki studies. The classes are also a chance to create community with other Reiki practitioners who share your goals.

Students have written to me after the classes to say how much more confidence they have in themselves and in Reiki, and that people who weren't interested before have started listening. The class discussions also helped students identify which skills they want to strengthen and how they might do so. The classes have been attended not only by lay Reiki practitioners, but also by physicians, nurses, physical therapists, and other health-care professionals who are Reiki practitioners. No one finds it easy to represent Reiki in words. However, there are learnable skills, information, and strategies that I have gleaned from years of medical and research collaboration that can help you bring Reiki into conventional medicine.

It is an exciting time to be a Reiki practitioner. We are literally creating the field of medical Reiki. We can be true to Reiki as a spiritual healing practice and help it become available to the mainstream public.

Reiki can be a humanizing factor in medicine that can facilitate the delivery of conventional care and support both patients and professionals. As patients and medical caregivers reach beyond the biomedical model to access the most complete health care possible, Reiki is a natural choice.

APPENDIX

SUGGESTED REIKI HAND PLACEMENTS

SUGGESTED HAND PLACEMENTS

These are the hand placements I use when giving a full treatment to myself or someone else, followed by additional placements you can use when sharing Reiki informally with a friend who is seated in a chair.

Let your hands be relaxed while giving Reiki treatment, just as if you were letting them rest comfortably on your lap, with the fingers neither spread widely apart nor squeezed together. When offering Reiki to someone else, hold your posture and avoid leaning on your friend.

The particular area of the body where you place your hands is more important than exactly how you place your hands there. For example, the illustrations show two options for placing your hands at your crown during self-treatment; you could also rest your head in your hands with your elbows on your desk, your lap or on pillows on your lap.

If you have any physical limitations, either acute or chronic, modify the placements as needed for your comfort and range of motion. You can use only one hand if necessary. If there are placements you are unable to reach, leave your hands longer at the placements you can reach with ease.

ABOUT YOUR POSTURE

Whether giving treatment to yourself or a friend, make yourself as comfortable as possible, adjusting your posture if you start to feel any discomfort. Avoid flexing your wrists, as they will quickly start to hurt. Keep them as long as possible, adjusting your posture if needed to do so. Also be careful not to torque your wrists or elbows or hyperextend your shoulders as you reach over your friend. Instead, find a way to sit closer.

For your own well-being—and at the risk of sounding like a yoga teacher—keep your pelvic sits bones planted on your chair, your spine long, and your shoulder blades moving slightly toward one another. Stay open across the upper chest and extended through the solar plexus area—don't round the spine or collapse into the stomach.

REIKI SELF-TREATMENT: SUGGESTED FULL PROTOCOL

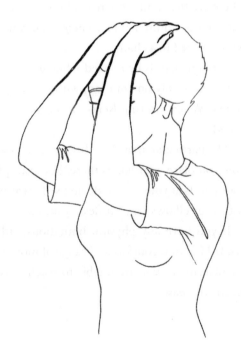

Front Crown

It's important that your hands cover the sensitive area at the very crown of your head, so keep your hands close to each other. Having your elbows in front usually works well, whether you are sitting or lying on your side (in which case you may want to place a pillow between your elbows).

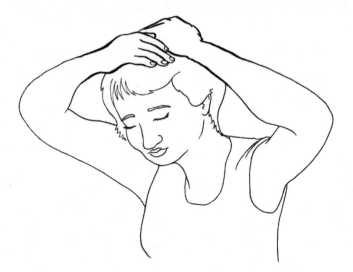

Sideways Crown
This approach can work whether you are sitting or lying on your back (again, support your arms with pillows as needed).

Face
Place your fingertips at your hairline and the heel of your hands on your cheekbones.

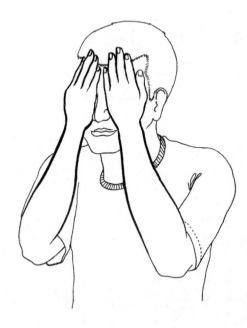

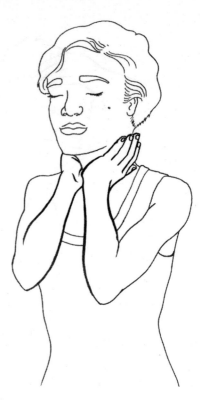

Throat

Place your fingers on the side of your neck and cup your palms over your larynx, with your wrists together.

Back of Head

Place your right hand above your left, with your hands side by side over the occipital ridge. Your hands are on the back of your skull, not the back of your neck.

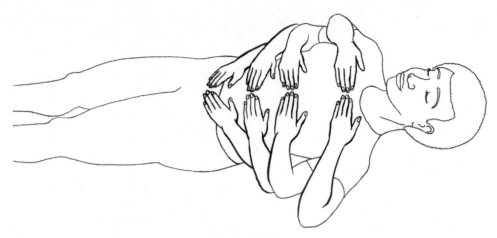

Front Torso

Place your hands on your upper chest, solar plexus, navel, and lower abdomen, successively, your fingertips close or even touching. Avoid overlapping your hands.

REIKI OTHER TREATMENT:
SUGGESTED FULL PROTOCOL

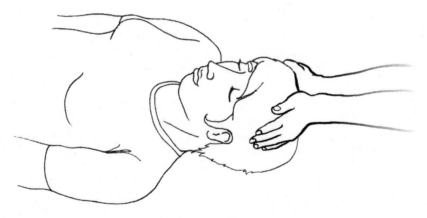

Crown Reiki

Sit behind your friend's head as she lies on her back. If you are able to place the heels of your hands together, you will be sure to cover the crown of her head. To do so, bring your elbows a little closer and rest them on pillows on your lap.

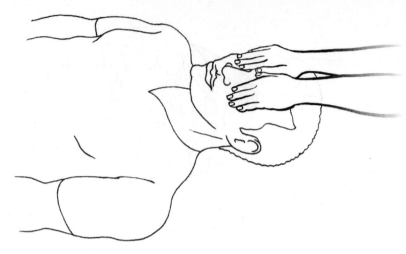

Face

Be mindful that you are touching someone's face. Place the heels of your hands at your friend's hair-line and rest your fingertips on his cheekbones. Avoid touching his lips or pinching his nostrils.

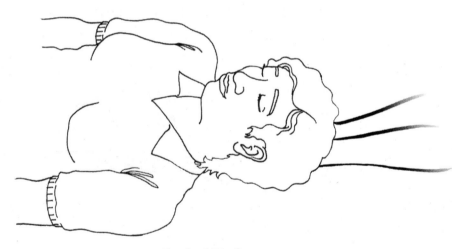

Back of Head

Rock your friend's head gently onto one hand and slip your other hand under her head. Rock her head into the palm of your first hand and place your second hand next to the first. The back of her head will rest in your palms as if they were made for each other.

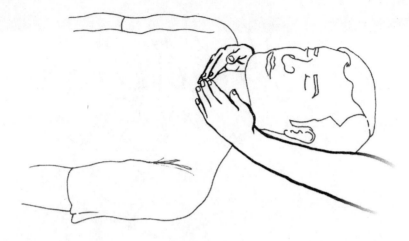

Throat

Many people are sensitive to being touched on the front of the throat. Resting your forearms on the treatment table, place your hands along the side of your friend's neck, touching his jaw or collarbones, and cupping your fingers over the front of his throat.

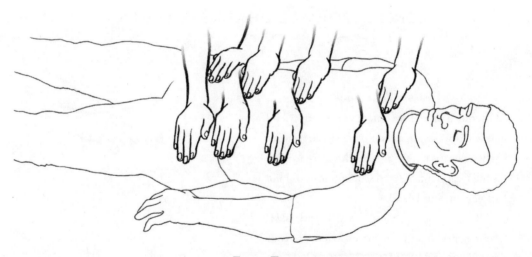

Front Torso

Be mindful of the central axis of the body. Place your hands close to each other on the upper three placements—upper chest, solar plexus, and navel. At the lower abdomen, move your hands farther apart, placing them over your friend's hip bones, so that your touch is not invasive.

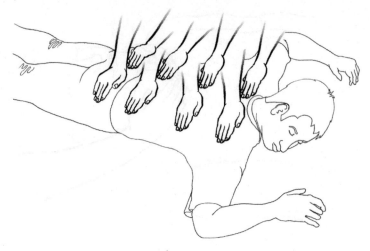

Back Torso

Again, be mindful of the body's central axis. Keep your hands close together as you place them on your friend's back, on his upper back, behind his heart, above his waist, and below his waist, at the sacrum.

REIKI INFORMAL CHAIR TREATMENT

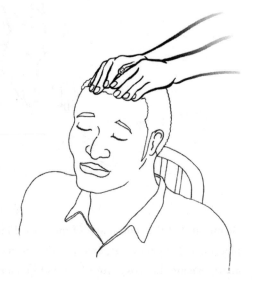

Crown (from back)

Offering a shorter treatment while your friend sits comfortably in a chair is a good alternative when there is not the time or the space to offer a full treatment. Stay present and mindful not to lean on your friend.

Standing behind your seated friend, place your hands lightly on his crown with your thumbs close or touching. (You could also do this from the side, which is not shown.)

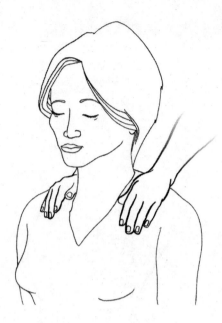

Shoulders (from back)

Standing or sitting behind your friend, place your hands comfortably on either shoulder.

Head (from side)

Standing or sitting at either side of your friend, place one of your hands on his forehead and the other hand at the occipital ridge on the back of his skull (it's the only ridge back there).

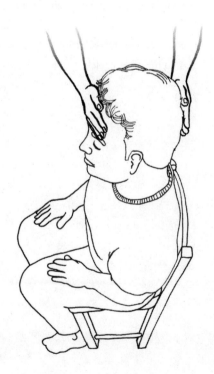

Upper Torso (from side)
While standing or sitting at your friend's side,
place one hand on her upper sternum, just below the notch of the collarbones, and the other
hand on her upper back.

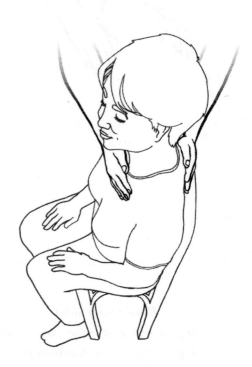

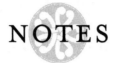

NOTES

Chapter One

1. http://nccam.nih.gov/health/backgrounds/energymed.htm#5.

2. R. O. Becker, "Acupuncture Points Show Increased DC Electrical Conductivity," *American Journal of Chinese Medicine,* 4 (1976): 69. M. Reichmanis, R. O. Becker, "Physiological Effects of Stimulation at Acupuncture Loci: A Review," *Comparative Medicine East and West,* 6 (1) (Spring 1978): 67–73. M. Reichmanis, A. A. Marino, R. O. Becker, "D.C. Skin Conductance Variation at Acupuncture Loci," *American Journal of Chinese Medicine,* 4 (1) (Spring 1976): 69–72. Research has shown acupuncture points have weaker resistance and correspondingly greater electrical conductivity than the surrounding skin. Perhaps the earliest scientist to study this was Robert O. Becker, M.D., an orthopedic surgeon and researcher twice nominated for the Nobel Prize in medicine. His first book, *The Body Electric* (1985), is devoted to electromagnetism and the human body, while his second book, *Cross Currents: The Promise of Electromedicine, The Perils of Electropollution* (1990), explains the scientific reasons behind his concern about the damaging effects caused by rapidly proliferating electromagnetic fields. Becker conducted NIH-funded research into the Chinese meridians as electrical conductors in the 1970s and is the author of numerous papers. A PubMed search of "Becker RO" brings up ninety titles published in peer-reviewed medical journals dating back to 1960. Becker graduated from New York University's medical school, was Professor of Medicine at NYU's Upstate Medical Center, and served as Director of Orthopedic Surgery at the Veterans Hospital in Syracuse for thirty years. Read more about his research on page 196.

Chapter Two

1. P. Miles, "Living in Relation to Mystery: Addressing Mind, Body, and Spirit," *Advances in Mind-Body Medicine,* 19 (2) (Summer 2003): 22–23.

2. A. C. Guyton and J. E. Hall, *Textbook of Medical Physiology,* 10th ed. (Saunders, 2000), chap. 1, p. 3. "To summarize, the body is actually *a social order of about 100 trillion cells* organized into different functional structures, some of which are called *organs*. Each functional structure provides its share in the maintenance of homeostatic conditions in the extracellular fluid, which is called the *internal environment*. As long as normal conditions are maintained in this internal environment, the cells of the body continue to live and function properly. Thus, each cell benefits from homeostasis, and in turn, each cell contributes its share toward the maintenance of homeostasis. This reciprocal interplay provides continuous automaticity of the body until one or more functional systems lose their ability to contribute their share of function. When this happens, all the cells of the body suffer. Extreme dysfunction leads to death, whereas moderate dysfunction leads to sickness" (author's italics).

3. C. N. Bernstein, A. Wajda, and J. F. Blanchard. "The Clustering of Other Chronic Inflammatory Diseases in Inflammatory Bowel Disease: A Population-Based Study," *Gastroenterology*, 129 (2005): 827–836.

4. G. Gupta, J. M. Gelfand, and J. D. Lewis, "Increased Risk of Demyelinating Diseases in Patients with Inflammatory Bowel Disease," *Gastroenterology* 129 (2005): 819–826.

5. T. K. V. Desikachar, *The Heart of Yoga: Developing a Personal Practice* (Rochester, VT: Inner Traditions, 1995), p. 59.

6. G. Deng and B. R. Cassileth, "Integrative Oncology: Complementary Therapies for Pain, Anxiety, and Mood Disturbance." *CA: A Cancer Journal for Clinicians,* 55 (2005): 109–116.

7. ". . . researchers are discovering that having a chronic illness can in fact enhance the way in which a patient engages with his or her life. It is thought that individuals can be transformed by the experience of living with chronic illness to experience positive outcomes." In A. L. Mulkins and M. J. Verhoef, "Supporting the Transformative Process: Experiences of Cancer Patients Receiving Integrative Care," *Integrative Cancer Therapies,* 3 (3) (2004): 1–8.

8. W. J. Kop, D. S. Krantz, B. D. Nearing, et al., "Effects of Acute Mental Stress and Exercise on T-Wave Alternans in Patients with Implantable Cardioverter Defibrilators and Controls," *Circulation,* 109 (15): (Apr. 20, 2004): 1864–1869; S. Koton, D. Tanne, N. M. Bornstein, and M. S. Green, "Triggering Risk Factors for Ischemic Stroke: A Case-Crossover Study," *Neurology,* 63 (Dec. 2004): 2006–2010.

9. J. P. van Melle, P. de Jonge, T. A. Spijkerman, et al., "Prognostic Association of Depression Following Myocardial Infarction with Mortality and Cardiovascular Events: A Meta-analysis," *Psychosomatic Medicine*, 66 (2004): 814–822; J. Barth, M. Schumacher, and C. Hermann-Lingen, "Depression as a Risk Factor for Mortality in Patients with Coronary Heart Disease: A Meta-analysis," *Psychosomatic Medicine,* 66 (2004): 802–13.

10. P. Miles, "Reiki for Mind, Body, and Spirit Support of Cancer Patients," *Advances in Mind-Body Medicine,* 22 (2) (Fall 2007). Open access at www.advancesjournal.com/adv/web_pdfs/miles.pdf.

11. M. L. Mingus, C. A. Bodian, C. N. Bradford, et al., "Prolonged Surgery Increases the Likelihood of Admission of Scheduled Ambulatory Surgery Patients," *Journal of Clinical Anesthesia,* 9 (1997): 446–450.
12. T. G. Monk, V. Saini, B. C. Weldon, and J. C. Sigl, "Anesthetic Management and One-Year Mortality After Noncardiac Surgery," *Anesthesia and Analgesia,* 100 (2005): 4–10.

Chapter Three

1. The Gakkai offers Reiju at each meeting to further expand the student's access to Reiki, but it is unclear if Usui had formalized this practice.
2. Hiroshi Doi, personal communication, April 2005.
3. H. Haberly, *Reiki: Hawayo Takata's Story* (Olney, MD: Archedigm, 1990), p. 18. Patsy Matsuura, "Mrs. Takata and Reiki Power," *Honolulu Advertiser*, February 25, 1974.
4. Vera Graham, "Universal Life Energy: Mrs. Takata Opens Minds to Reiki," *San Mateo County Times,* May 17, 1975.
5. Haberly, *Reiki: Hawayao Takata's Story,* p. 20.
6. Graham, "Universal Life Energy."
7. Fran Brown, *Living Reiki: Takata's Teachings* (Mendocino, CA: LifeRhythm, 1992), p. 27.
8. Paul Prakash Dennis, personal communication, August 16, 2005.
9. Wanja Twan, personal communication, April 2, 2003.
10. Paul Prakash Dennis, personal communication, August 16, 2005.
11. *Reiki Magazine International,* "First Person: Mrs. Takata Tells Her Story: Cause and Effect," 3 (1): 8.
12. www.robertfueston.com.
13. Anneli Twan, *Early Days of Reiki: Memories of Hawayo Takata* (Hope, British Columbia: Morning Star Productions, 2005), p. 13.

Chapter Four

1. Haberly, *Reiki: Hawayo Takata's Story,* p. 59.

Chapter Five

1. You can also call (208) 783-4848, or write to the Reiki Alliance at 204 North Chestnut Street, Kellogg, ID 83837.

Chapter Six

1. Haberly, *Reiki: Hawayo Takata's Story,* p. 51.
2. Paul Mitchell and Susan Mitchell, personal communication.
3. Haberly, *Reiki: Hawayo Takata's Story,* p. 59.
4. www.reikialliance.com.
5. Kurt Kaltreider, *American Indian Prophecies: Conversations with Chasing Deer* (Carlsbad, CA: Hay

House, 1998). Also, Kurt Kaltreider, *American Indian Cultural Heroes and Teaching Tales* (Carlsbad, CA: Hay House, 2004).

6. Charles F. Finch III, "African Medicine: Emerging from the Shadows," *Proceedings of the Fourth Annual Alternative Therapies Symposium,* New York City, March 25–28, 1999, p. 136.

Chapter Seven

1. When prayer specifically for health was included as a CAM intervention, 63 percent of the respondents to the 2002 National Health Interview Survey conducted by the Centers for Disease Control and Prevention's (CDC) National Center for Health Statistics used CAM in the previous twelve months. Forty-three percent used prayer for their own health, 24.4 percent had others pray for their health, and 9.6 percent participated in prayer groups to pray for their health. When prayer was excluded, respondents using CAM dropped to 36 percent.

2. According to Kenneth Cohen, author *The Way of Qigong: The Art and Science of Chinese Energy Healing* and *Honoring the Medicine,* the use of symbols was common in Taoist healing. Japanese culture at the time was permeated by three main spiritual influences, Buddhism, Taoism, and Shintoism. Personal communication, Dec. 26, 2002.

3. Hiroshi Doi, personal communication, April 2005.

4. John Snelling, *The Buddhist Handbook: A Complete Guide to Buddhist Schools, Teaching, Practice, and History* (Rochester, VT: Inner Traditions, 1991), p. 99.

Chapter Eight

1. Twan, *Early Days of Reiki,* p. 39.
2. Haberly, *Reiki: Hawayo Takata's Story,* p. 51.

Chapter Nine

1. Twan, *Early Days of Reiki,* p. 12.
2. Haberly, *Reiki: Hawayo Takata's Story,* p. 58.
3. Brown, *Living Reiki: Takata's Teachings,* p. 69
4. Kausthub Desikachar, personal communication, May 5, 2004.

Chapter Ten

1. B. R. H. Van den Bergh and A. Marcoen, "High Antenatal Maternal Anxiety is Related to ADHA Symptoms, Externalizing Problems and Anxiety in 8- and 9-Year-Olds," *Child Development,* 75 (4) (July 2004): 1085–1097; R. E. Tremblay, D. S. Nagin, J. R. Seguin, et al., "Physical Aggression During Early Childhood: Trajectories and Predictors," *Pediatrics,* 114 (2004): e43–e50.

2. R. M. Sapolsky, "Mothering Style and Methylation," *Nature Neuroscience,* 7 (Aug. 2004): 791–792; I. C. G.

Weaver, N. Cervoni, F. A. Champagne, et al., "Epigenetic Programming by Maternal Behavior," *Nature Neuroscience,* 7 (2004): 847–854.

3. Haberly, *Reiki: Hawayo Takata's Story,* p. 67.

4. L. S. Lohmander, A. Ostenberg, M. Englund, and H. Roos, "High Prevalence of Knee Osteoarthritis, Pain, and Functional Limitations in Female Soccer Players Twelve Years After Anterior Cruciate Ligament Injury," *Arthritis & Rheumatism,* 50 (10) (2004): 3145–3152.

5. Richard J. Davidson, Ph.D., director of W. M. Keck Laboratory of Functional Brain Imaging and Behavior at the University of Wisconsin, Madison, is widely acknowledged to be the founder of affective neuroscience. People experiencing negative emotional states have less activity in the left prefrontal cortex and more in the right. Davidson's research showed that meditation increases activity in the left prefrontal cortex, even in beginners, and links this with increased immunity. R. J. Davidson, J. Kabat-Zinn, J. Schumacher, M. Rosenkranz, D. Muller, S. F. Santorelli, F. Urbanowski, A. Harrington, K. Bonus, and J. F. Sheridan, "Alterations in Brain and Immune Function Produced by Mindfulness Meditation," *Psychosomatic Medicine,* 65 (2003): 564–570.

6. *Reiki Magazine International,* 5 (3) (June/July 2003): 35.

7. For more information, contact the National Institute on Aging Information Center, PO Box 8057, Gaithersburg, MD 20898-8057; 1-800-222-2225, 1-800-222-4225 (TTY); www.nia.nih.gov.

8. K. M. Langa, M. A. Valenstein, A. M. Fendrick, M. U. Kabeto, S. Vijan, "Extent and Cost of Informal Caregiving for Older Americans with Symptoms of Depression," *American Journal of Psychiatry,* 161 (5) (May 2004): 857–863.

9. http://www.mentalhealth.samhsa.gov/suicideprevention/elderly.asp (accessed Sept. 10, 2005).

10. T. M. Gill, H. G. Allore, T. R. Holford, and Z. Guo, "Hospitalization, Restricted Activity, and the Development of Disability Among Older Persons," *Journal of the American Medical Association,* 292 (2004): 2115–2124.

Chapter Eleven

1. D. M. Eisenberg, R. C. Kessler, C. Foster, F. E. Norlock, D. R. Calkins, and T. L. Delbanco. "Unconventional Medicine in the United States. Prevalence, Costs, and Patterns of Use," *New England Journal of Medicine,* 328 (4) (Jan. 28, 1993): 246–52; D. M. Eisenberg, R. B. Davis, S. L. Ettner, S. Appel, S. Wilkey, M. Van Rompay, and R. C. Kessler, "Trends in Alternative Medicine Use in the United States, 1990–1997: Results of a Follow-up National Survey," *Journal of the American Medical Association,* 280 (1998): 1569–1575.

2. P. Miles, "Reiki for Mind, Body, and Spirit Support of Cancer Patients," *Advances in Mind-Body Medicine,* 22 (2) (Fall 2007). Open access at www.advancesjournal.com/adv/web_pdfs/miles.pdf.

3. P. Miles, "If There Is Any Significant Experience with Using Reiki in the Hospital or ER Setting and If There Is Any Literature to Support This Use?" *Explore,* 1 (5): 414 (Sept. 2005).

4. P. Bailey, "Code Blue: Healing Touch," *Hospital Physician,* 33 (1) (1997): 42.

Chapter Twelve

1. Haberly, *Reiki: Hawayo Takata's Story,* p. 27.

2. D. M. Eisenberg et al., "Unconventional Medicine," 246–52.

3. L. Capasso, *Lancet,* 352 (9143) (December 5, 1998): 1864.

4. Charles S. Finch III, personal communication, March 28, 1999.

5. D. M. Eisenberg et al., "Trends in Alternative Medicine Use," 1569–1575.

6. Kaltreider, *American Indian Prophecies* and *American Indian Cultural Heroes;* Jean Liedloff, *The Continuum Concept: In Search of Happiness Lost* (Da Capo Press, 1986), 1975.

7. Chukuka Enwemeka, Ph.D., PT, observes that tissue repair is not cerebral intelligence, yet his research has documented a complex and predictable process of cellular scattering and reorganization in the healing process of severed rabbit tendons. He comments further that the fact that the very strong Achilles tendon ruptures while lesser tendons remain intact points to the existence of an underlying pathology that is weakening the tendon. Personal communication, February 9, 2005.

8. A. P. Beltrami, K. Urbanek, J. Kajstura, et al., "Evidence That Human Cardiac Myocytes Divide After Myocardial Infarction," *New England Journal of Medicine,* 344 (23) (June 7, 2001): 1750–1757; and personal communication, February 15, 2005.

9. James L. Oschman, Ph.D., personal communication, January 3, 2005.

10. Daniel Odier, *Yoga Spandakarika: The Sacred Texts at the Origins of Tantra* (Rochester, VT: Inner Traditions, 2005); Jayadev Singh, *Spanda Karikas: The Divine Creative Pulsation* (Benares, India: Motilal Banarsidass Publishers, 1994); Mark S. G. Dyczkowski, *The Doctrine of Vibration* (Albany: SUNY Press, 1987); Jayadev Singh, trans., Ksemaraja, *Doctrine of Self-Recognition: A Translation of the Pratyabhinjnahrdayam* (Albany: SUNY Press, 1990); Mark S. G. Dyczkowski, trans. Vasugupta, *The Stanzas on Vibration: The Spandakarika with Four Commentaries: The Spandasamdoha by Ksemaraja, the Spandavrtti by Kallatabhatta, the Spandavivr* (Albany: SUNY Press, 1992); Guenther H. Longchenpa, *Kindly Bent to Ease Us* (Berkeley, CA: Dharma Publishing, 1976); David Snellgrove, *The Hevajra Tantra: A Critical Study*, London Oriental Series, vol. 6 (Oxford University Press, 1980).

11. M. F. Green and M. Kinsbourne, "Auditory Hallucinations in Schizophrenia: Does Humming Help?" *Biological Psychiatry,* 27 (8) (1990): 934–935.

12. M. Maniscalco, M. Sofia, E. Weitzbert, L. Arratu, and J. O. Lundberg, "Nasal Nitric Oxide Measurements Before and After Repeated Humming Maneuvers." *European Journal of Clinical Investigation,* 33 (12) (2003): 1090–1094.

13. E. Weitzberg, J. O. Lundberg. "Humming Greatly Increases Nasal Nitric Oxide," *American Journal of Respiratory and Critical Care Medicine,* 166 (2) (2002): 131–132.

14. T. G. Monk, V. Saini, B. Weldon, and J. C. Sigl, "Anesthetic Management and One-Year Mortality after Noncardiac Surgery," *Anesthesia and Analgesia,* 100 (2005): 4–10.

Chapter Thirteen

1. Andrew Weil, M.D., pesonal communication, January 5, 2005.

2. A number of peer-reviewed medical papers articulate the challenges of researching complementary therapies from a balanced, informed perspective, and offer valuable insights to guide the creation of meaningful, credible CAM research: K. I. Block, A. J. Cohen, A. S. Dobs, D. Ornish, D. Tripathy, "The Challenges of Randomized Trials in Integrative Cancer Care," *Integrative Cancer Therapies,* 3 (2) (June 2004): 112–27; I. R. Bell, O. Caspi, G. E. R. Schwartz, K. L. Grant, T. W. Gaudet, D. Rychener, V. Maizes, and A. Weil, "Integrative Medicine and Systemic Outcomes Research; Issues in the Emergence of a New Model for Primary Health Care," *Archives of Internal Medicine,* 162 (2002): 133–40; K. J. Kemper, B. R. Cassileth, and T. Ferris, "Holistic Pediatrics: A Research Agenda," *Pediatrics,* 103 (1999): 902–9; H. Walach, W. B. Jonas, and G. T. Lewith, "The Role of Outcomes Research in Evaluating Complementary and Alternative Medicines," *Alternative Therapies in Health and Medicine,* 8 (3) (May/June 2002): 88–95; O. Caspi and K. O. Burleson, "Methodological Challenges in Meditation Research," *Advances in Mind-Body Medicine,* 21 (1) (Spring 2005): 4–11; L. Mehl-Madrona, "Connectivity and Healing: Some Hypotheses about the Phenomenon and How to Study It," *Advances in Mind-Body Medicine,* 21(1) (Spring 2005): 12–28.

3. P. Miles and G. True, "Reiki: Review of a Biofield Therapy History, Theory, Practice, and Research," *Alternative Therapies in Health and Medicine,* 9 (2) (March/April 2003): 62–72. P. Miles, "Reiki for Mind, Body, and Spirit Support of Cancer Patients," *Advances in Mind-Body Medicine,* 22 (2) (Fall 2007). The research section includes a couple of interesting studies published after the review. Open access at www.advances.journal.com/adv/web_pdfs/miles/pdf.

4. http://clinicaltrials.gov/search/term=(NCCAM)+%5BSPONSOR%5D+(reiki)+%5BTREATMENT% 5D?recruiting=false. Accessed January 2, 2008.

5. D. W. Wardell and J. Engebretson, "Biological Correlates of Reiki Touch Healing," *Journal of Advanced Nursing,* 33 (4) (2001): 439–45.

6. N. Mackay, S. Hansen, O. McFarlane, "Autonomic Nervous Systems During Reiki Treatment: A Preliminary Study," *Journal of Alternative and Complementary Medicine,* 10 (6) (Dec. 2004): 1077–1081.

7. K. Olson, J. Hanson, and M. Michaud, "A Phase II Trial of Reiki for the Management of Pain in Advanced Cancer Patients," *Journal of Pain Symptom Management,* 26 (5) (Nov. 2003): 990–997.

8. P. Miles, "Reiki for Mind, Body, and Spirit Support of Cancer Patients," *Advances in Mind-Body Medicine,* 22 (2) (Fall 2007). The research section includes a couple of interesting studies published after the review. Open access at www.advancesjournal.com/adv/web_pdfs/miles/pdf.

9. K. L. Tsand, L. E. Carlson, and K. Olson, "Pilot Crossover Trial of Reiki Versus Rest for Treating Cancer-Related Fatigue," *Integrative Cancer Therapies,* 6 (1) (2007) 25–35.

10. A. Vitale and P. C. O'Connor. "The Effect of Reiki on Pain and Anxiety on Women with Abdominal Hysterectomies: A Quasi-Experimental Pilot Study," *Holistic Nursing Practice,* 20 (6) (2006): 263–272.

11. This was a simple study that could easily be replicated in other populations. The STAI State-Trait Anxi-

ety Scale can be purchased from Charles D. Spielberger at http://www.mindgarden.com/products/staisad.htm.

12. P. Miles, "Preliminary Report on the Use of Reiki for HIV-Related Pain and Anxiety," *Alternative Therapies in Health and Medicine,* 9 (2) (March/April 2003): 36.

13. J. Engebretson and D. Wardell, "Experience of a Reiki Session," *Alternative Therapies in Health and Medicine,* 8 (200): 48–53.

14. A. G. Shore, "Long-Term Effects of Energetic Healing on Symptoms of Psychological Depression and Self-Perceived Stress," *Alternative Therapies in Health and Medicine,* 10 (3) (May–June 2004): 42–48.

15. B. R. Cassileth and A. J. Vickers, "Massage Therapy for Symptom Control: Outcome Study at a Major Cancer Center," *Journal of Pain Symptom Management,* 28 (3) (2004): 244–49.

16. H. Moses, E. R. Dorsey, D. H. M. Matheson, S. O. Thier, "Financial Anatomy of Biomedical Research," *Journal of the American Medical Association,* 294 (2005): 1333–1342.

Chapter Fourteen

1. D. M. Eisenberg, R. C. Kessler, C. Foster, F. E. Norlock, D. R. Calkins, and T. L. Delbanco, "Unconventional Medicine in the United States: Prevalence, Costs, and Patterns of Use." *New England Journal of Medicine,* 328 (4) (Jan. 28, 1993): 246–252.

2. According to this paper, "energy healing" was one of the categories of therapy that increased most in usage from the survey in 1990 to the one in 1997, and the authors specifically named Reiki as being reported under the category "energy medicine." D. M. Eisenberg, R. B. Davis, S. L. Ettner, et al., "Trends in Alternative Medicine Use in the United States, 1990–1997: Results of a Follow-up National Survey," *Journal of the American Medical Association,* 280 (1998): 1569–1575.

3. In a survey by the Centers for Disease Control, adding prayer specifically for one's own health increased the percentage of respondents to who used CAM within the past twelve months from 36 to 62 percent. As in the 1998 paper by Eisenberg et al., Reiki is listed with "energy medicine." P. M. Barnes, E. Powell-Griner, K. McFann, and R. L. Nahin, "Complementary and Alternative Medicine Use Among Adults: United States, 2002," *CDC Advance Data Report,* no. 343 (2004).

4. J. A. Astin, "Why Patients Use Alternative Medicine: Results of a National Study." *Journal of the American Medical Association,* 279 (1998): 1548–53.

5. Patients who chose a physician associated with CAM, or an alternative practitioner (chiropractor, naturopath, or homeopath) for their direct health care scored higher on a psychospiritual testing instrument (SIBS) than did those who chose a conventional physician. J. J. Petry and R. Finkel, "Spirituality and Choice of Health Care Practitioner," *Journal of Alternative and Complementary Medicine* 10 (6) (2004): 939–45.

6. B. L. Wellman, M. Kelner, and B. Wigdor, "Older Adults' Use of Medical and Alternative Care," *Journal of Applied Gerontology* 20 (1) (March 2001): 3–23.

7. J. Dalen, "Conventional and Unconventional: Can They Be Integrated?" *Archives of Internal Medicine,* 158: 2179–2181.

8. *The Yellow Emperor's Classic of Medicine,* trans. Maoshing Ni (Boston: Shambala, 1995), p. 7.

9. Schmehr published a case report documenting the benefits of one clinic patient who cites Reiki as "the single greatest factor contributing to his successful behavior change" in overcoming depression, cocaine addiction, poverty, and an unwillingness to be a responsible partner in his health care. Seven years after learning Reiki, now seventy years old, the patient is receiving international acclaim for the art he has created since learning Reiki. He relishes his daily practice, attributing to it not only emotional, behavioral, and physical benefits, but a profound expansion of his creativity. R. Schmehr, "Enhancing Treatment of HIV/AIDS with Reiki Training and Treatment," *Alternative Therapies in Health and Medicine,* 9 (2) (March/April 2003): 118, 120.

10. M. H. Cohen, D. M. Eisenberg, "Potential Physician Malpractice Liability Associated with Complementary and Integrative Medical Therapies," *Annals of Internal Medicine,* 136 (2002): 596.

11. The Touch Research Institute of the University of Miami School of Medicine has been researching the effects of massage therapy on various functions and medical conditions since 1992 under the direction of Tiffany Field, Ph.D. The website www.miami.edu/touch-research/ lists more than ninety studies showing benefits such as diminished pain with fibromyalgia, reduced occurrence of autoimmune function, and improved alertness and performance. Many of these benefits are thought to be attributable to decreased stress hormones. Monthly two-day workshops on conducting touch research are offered.

12. The Program in Integrative Medicine (PIM) at the University of Arizona offers online courses, associate and residential fellowships, one-month rotations for medical students and residents, and conferences on botanical medicine, integrative pain medicine, and nutrition and health. The website www.integrative medicine.arizona.edu lists PIM physician graduates by location.

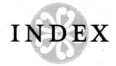

INDEX

ABOUT THE AUTHOR

Pamela Miles, an integrative health-care consultant and Reiki master with thirty-five years' experience in natural healing, has been practicing Reiki since 1986. She has created Reiki programs in New York City hospitals, collaborated in various clinical and research settings (infectious disease, cancer, surgery, ICU, organ transplantation, rehab, labor and delivery, hospice) and taught Reiki to medical staff and students. In her private practice, Miles has worked with people addressing a wide range of conditions, including heart disease, cancer, HIV, sickle-cell anemia, asthma, autism, MS, lupus, CP, fatigue syndromes, IBS, Crohn's disease, stroke, infertility, ADD and ADHD, and Lyme disease, as well as advising healthy people who wish to strengthen their well-being. She is the founding director of the Institute for the Advancement of Complementary Therapies (I*ACT) and has published articles in peer-reviewed medical journals and popular magazines, many of which are available at www.ReikiInMedicine.org. Miles conducts trainings for Reiki students and practitioners to prepare for professional practice and medical collaboration.